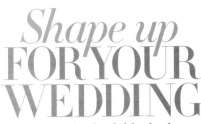

Shape up FOR YOUR WEDDING

The complete bridal-body plan

Health&Fitness MAGAZINE

Words Joanna Ebsworth
Photography Ian Derry
Models Georgia @ Milk Management, Lara Raybone @ W Athletic
Clothing credits Coast Darling Dress, £295 (coast-stores.com).
The Way You Look Tonight tiara, price on request (irresistibleheaddresses.com)
Ring, £256 (brilliantinc.co.uk)
Stylist Kellie Daggett
Hair & make-up Claire Portman

Editor Mary Comber
Sub-editors Eve Boggenpoel, Emma Lewis, Charlie Jackson
Art editor Laura Passmore
Designer Jo Elston

MagBook publisher Dharmesh Mistry
Digitial production manager Nicky Baker
Operations director Robin Ryan
MagBook account manager Katie Wood
Managing director of advertising Julian Lloyd-Evans
Newstrade director David Barker
Retail & commercial director Martin Belson
Publisher Nicola Bates
Group publisher Russell Blackman
Group managing director Ian Westwood
Chief operating officer Brett Reynolds
Group finance director Ian Leggett
Chief executive James Tye
Chairman Felix Dennis

MAGBOOK

Shape Up Yor Your Wedding ISBN 1-78106-093-2

To license this product, contact Carlotta Serantoni, +44 (0) 20 7907 6550, carlotta_serantoni@dennis.co.uk.
To syndicate this content, contact Anj Dosaj-Halai, +44 (0)20 7907 6132, anj_dosaj-halai@dennis.co.uk.

Contents

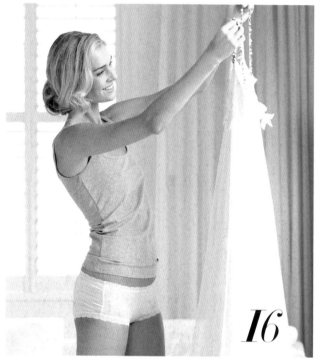

16

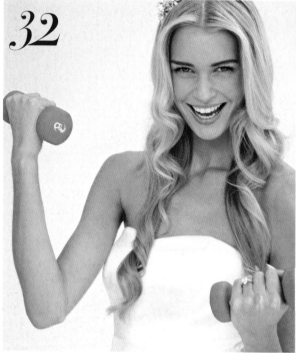

32

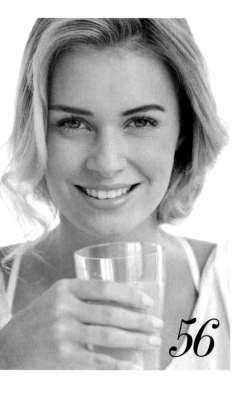

56

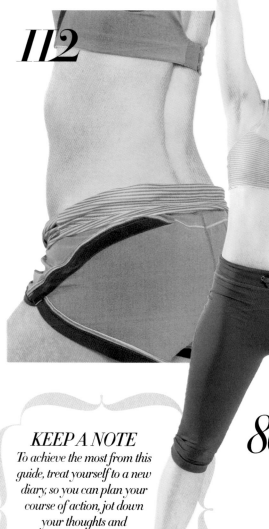

112

86

KEEP A NOTE
To achieve the most from this guide, treat yourself to a new diary, so you can plan your course of action, jot down your thoughts and inspirations, record test results and monitor your progress as your big day approaches.

CHANGE

YOUR REFLECTION

Diet Protein™ is arguably the most sophisticated diet protein shake available today. Reflex Nutrition have used the latest advances in protein and weight loss science to bring you a product that's specifically designed to help you achieve a healthy, well defined and toned body.

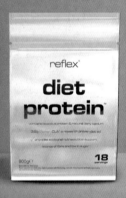

RRP £32.99
900g - 18 x 50g servings

There are many surveys published analyzing the CLA (conjugated linoleic acid) content of foods from around the world which show that intake of CLA is lower than in scientific studies where beneficial health effects are induced.

Research also suggests that in order to obtain the reported health benefits of CLA, supplementation is required.

Reflex Diet Protein™ is the only sports supplement available today that uses a 3.2g daily dose of CLA which is substantiated as an effective dose by research.

Each serving of Reflex Diet Protein™ is packed with additional diet support. Green Tea extract is added for its long standing reputation for aiding dieters.

Diet Protein™ contains no added sugar or maltodextrin. It's perfect for dieters wanting to restrict their carbohydrate content.

Diet Protein™ comes in a variety of mouthwatering flavours, all of which have been up against a taste test panel to ensure that they are the best tasting diet shakes on the market.

Find out more about our products at:

www.reflex-nutrition.com

 Please visit & join our Facebook page at Reflex Nutrition Ltd   @ReflexNutrition   ecotricity

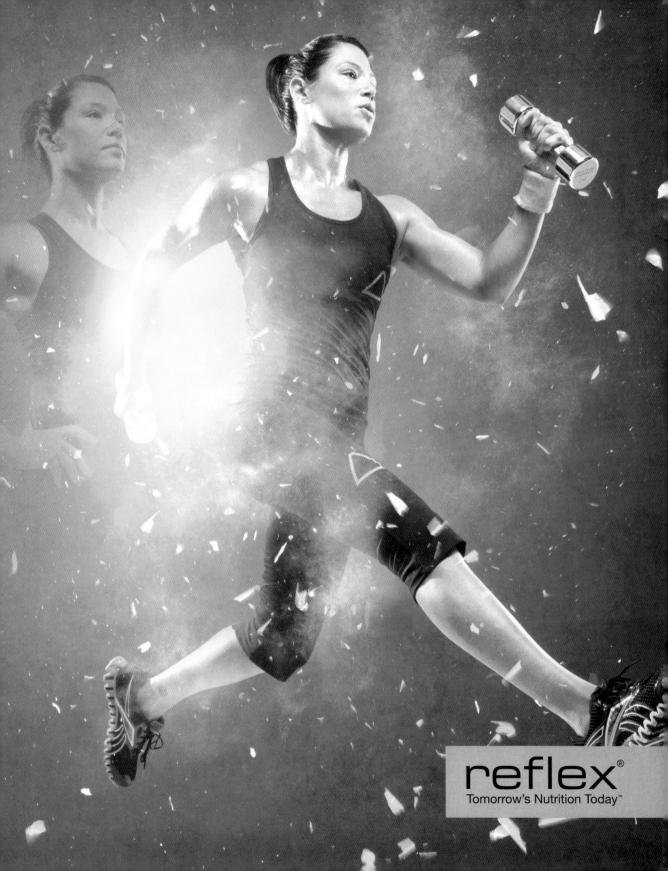

reflex®
Tomorrow's Nutrition Today™

About the author

JOANNA EBSWORTH is a top women's fitness and weight-loss expert. With over 10 years' experience in the health and fitness industry, she splits her time between training her female-only clients and writing for some of the UK's most respected publications including *Health & Fitness* magazine. Jo's helped hundreds of women lose weight, tone up and lead healthier lifestyles with her fun and effective workouts — including dozens of brides who want to look their best ever!

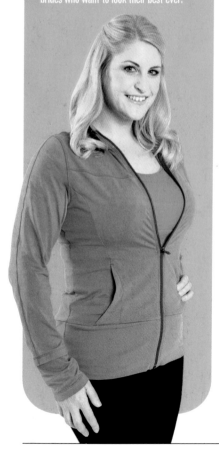

Just got engaged? Congratulations!

Don't know where to start getting the body of your dreams for the big day? Fear not! You are now holding perhaps the best engagement present you could give yourself – an in-depth guide written especially for brides-to-be that reveals everything you need to know about getting into the best shape of your life.

Planning a wedding is one of the most exciting things you can do, but with it comes a huge amount of pressure, especially when you're trying to lose weight and tone up at the same time. So to help you start planning and implementing your transformation, I've put together all the essential information you need to take the stress out of looking slim and stunning, from eating your way to gorgeous skin, nails and hair and appearing instantly slimmer with better posture, to finding the perfect dress to flatter your shape so you look amazing in your wedding photos. You'll also find a six-week workout plan packed with safe yet highly effective exercises (many used by your favourite A-list celebrities) to help you torch calories, work muscles you never knew you had and banish your trouble zones for a slender yet beautifully sculpted bridal body.

When you think of the word bride, the words blushing, beautiful and radiant come to mind, not tired, stressed or scrawny. That's why you won't find any quick-fix starvation diets or drastic exercise regimes in this book – just lots of sensible expert advice that will help you adopt positive exercise and healthy eating habits you can maintain long after you say your vows. And don't forget, we'll be here every step of the way to help motivate and inspire you on your journey as you work towards leading a fitter, healthier and happier life.

Get ready to say 'I do' to a whole new slimmer and more beautiful you!

Joanna

JOANNA EBSWORTH
Personal trainer; jo2go.co.uk

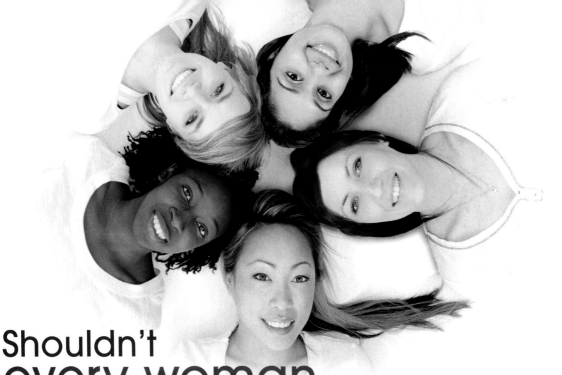

Shouldn't every woman be a *wellwoman*?

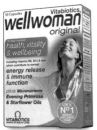
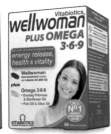
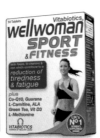
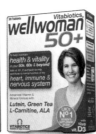
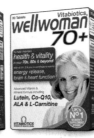
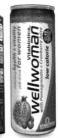
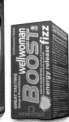

The UK's No. 1 supplements for women's health

Whether you are looking to support general daily health or have a specific health interest, the *Vitabiotics Wellwoman® range* offers an advanced range of nutritional products designed to safeguard your nutritional intake and life stage needs. With 40 years experience, there's no women's supplement range more relied on than Vitabiotics Wellwoman®.

Originally developed with

Prof. A. H. Beckett†
OBE, PhD, DSc
(1920-2010)
Professor Emeritus,
University of London

Wellwoman supports

From , Superdrug, Holland & Barrett, Lloydspharmacy, GNC, supermarkets, health stores, independent pharmacies & **www.vitabiotics.com**

Vitamin supplements may benefit those with nutritionally inadequate diets.
† Professor Beckett is not cited in the capacity of a health professional, but as a product inventor and former Chairman of Vitabiotics.

Britain's leading
supplements
for specific life stages

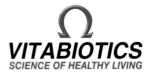
VITABIOTICS
SCIENCE OF HEALTHY LIVING

How to USE THIS BOOK

We'll be with you every step of the way, as you plan your perfect wedding

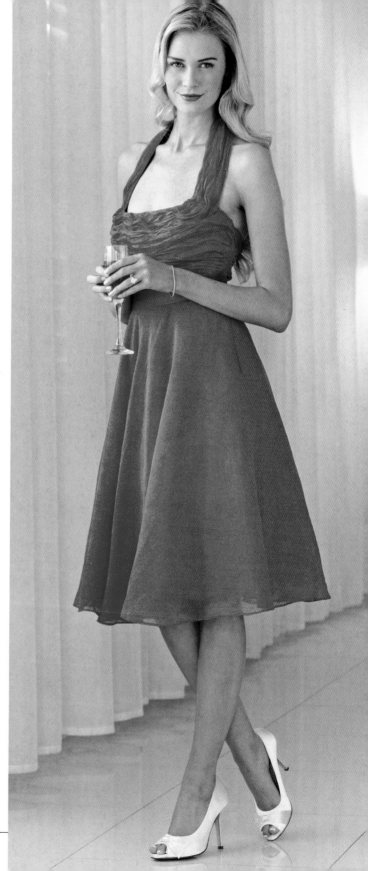

CLOTHING: Dress, £135 (coast-stores.com). Princess bracelet, £135 and ring, £295 (brilliant.co.uk). Sasso shoes, £140 (rainbowclub.com)

T he secret of looking beautiful on your big day is down to several factors, including a healthy diet, regular exercise, great grooming and self-belief. You might be tempted to turn straight to the workouts so you can start toning your body right away, but we suggest reading the guide from cover to cover first. This way you'll get an overview of the path to your bridal transformation. You'll benefit along the way from tips and tricks to instantly boost your figure and confidence, find out how to eat well for more energy and take tests to establish your fitness levels and exercise personality, so you know which type of exercise will work best for you – all the ingredients you need for a fulfilling and successful journey to becoming a beautiful bride.

Boost your confidence

Looking good starts with feeling good, so first of all we'll show you how to exude beauty from the inside out. Turn to 'Body confidence' (pages 14-29) for your guide to feeling more positive about yourself, getting perfect posture to radiate confidence and poise, beating stress to keep calm and healthy, and finding the perfect wedding dress for your body shape.

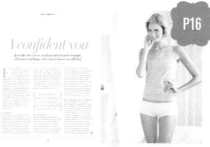

Prepare to get fit

Discover the amazing benefits of exercise in 'Get in shape' (pages 30-49). Take our health MOT and fitness tests to establish your entry level to the workouts, and discover your fitness personality with our quiz. You'll also find a pick of the best bridal bootcamps (and tips to survive them), plus advice on how to get fit with your man – and for the bedroom!

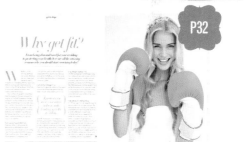

Eat yourself beautiful

If you want to lose weight, have bags of energy and healthy hair, skin and nails, you need the right nutrients. Take our nutrition test in the 'Slim & healthy' section (pages 50-65) to see how good (or bad) your diet is and what areas you can improve. Then check out the foods to eat for optimum health, plus those that sabotage your weight-loss efforts.

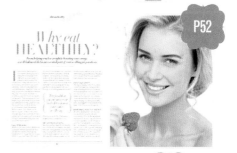

Natural beauty

Getting pampered and preened is one of the most enjoyable parts of prepping for your wedding. The 'Beautiful you' section (pages 66-79) shows you how to get lustrous locks and glowing skin, optimise your looks with clever grooming tricks and, most importantly, avoid any potential beauty disasters before your big day arrives.

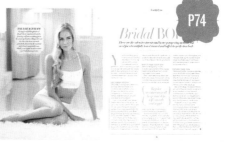

Your six-week plan

It's time to work up a sweat, with 'The Workouts' section (pages 80-125). As well as the full-body routine, six mini-plans target the trouble zones all brides worry about, including bingo wings, muffin tops and saddle bags. There's also a six-week plan to guide you through your shape-up regime, and progress charts to help you monitor your results. ≫

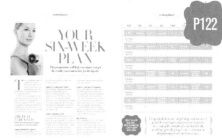

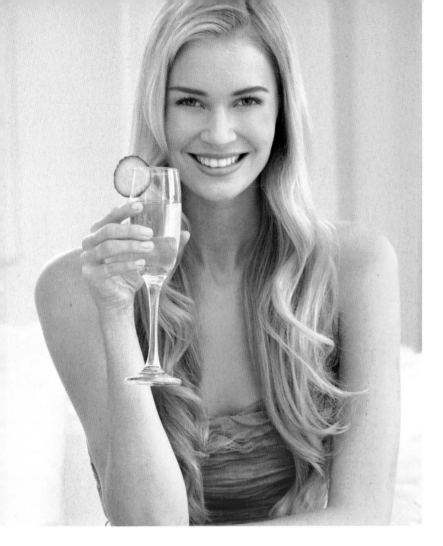

Time to PLAN

Be 100 per cent beautiful on your big day with this handy countdown. Whether you have 10 months or 10 weeks to go, there's always something you can do to make the day extra special

Twelve months to go...
DITCH THE TOXINS

Because it takes a while for your body to get rid of built-up toxins, you need to think about cutting down on sugar, caffeine and alcohol, so your skin and eyes sparkle on the big day. Clear all the junk food from your house to help you to avoid temptations that can set you back and cause you extra stress.

Eleven months to go...
BRIDESMAID BONDING

Once you've selected the lucky few to share the journey with you, start some social fitness challenges with your bridesmaids to keep you all motivated. Think Zumba classes (zumba.com), hot yoga (bikramyoga.co.uk) and long walks, where you can discuss all your big plans while getting fit at the same time.

Ten months to go...
BOOK YOUR BOOTCAMP

If you think you'll need a bootcamp retreat to hit your target weight, now's the time to book. You can lose up to 10lbs in a week (depending on how much you have to lose in the first place) so you'll want to go sooner rather than later, and definitely before you start trying on wedding dresses, as your body shape can dramatically change.

Nine months to go...
WEDDING DRESS SHOPPING

Start researching what style will complement your shape and then work out which areas you'll need to tone up before your dress fittings begin. If you're hoping for major weight loss, resist ordering a dress at this time no matter how excited you get or if you spot a bargain – you could end up spending a small fortune on alterations, or even on another dress!

Eight months to go...
TIME TO GET FIT

If you haven't already introduced some regular fitness into your life, now's the time. Aim for at least three workout sessions a week, so you don't find yourself in a blind shape-up panic a few weeks before the wedding. Also, start increasing your daily moderate activity levels (find out more on page 35).

Seven months to go...
BRIDAL BEAUTY PREP

It's a good idea to get serious about your skincare early on. Start a good cleansing and moisturising programme for your face, and consider making appointments for monthly facials to help replenish your skin and target problem areas. Regular body-brushing, exfoliating and moisturising in earnest will help reduce cellulite, boost skin tone and give you silky soft skin. Use a nourishing hair treatment once a week.

Four months to go...
BOOK HAIR AND MAKE-UP TRIALS

Be organised and take pictures of make-up trends and hairstyles you like and any accessories you plan to wear. If you've been thinking about drastically cutting or colouring your hair, book two or three appointments now (six to eight weeks apart) so you can get the perfect shade and style for your wedding.

> 'Start some social fitness challenges with your bridesmaids, to help motivation'

Three months to go...
TANNING TEST-OUT

If you're planning on having a spray tan for the big day, start trying out local therapists to find the right one (and colour!) for you. If you're going to self-tan, it's best to experiment with different products and application methods now, to avoid any tanning disasters for the day itself.

Two months to go...
FINAL WEIGHT LOSS

It's crunch time. If you want your dress to fit you really well, then you need to focus on your diet, and banish any bad habits. If you're too stressed to think about making healthy packed lunches, sign up for a home delivery service, such as Pure Package (purepackage.com) or Soulmatefood (soulmatefood.com).

Four weeks before...
TIME TO TONE UP

This is it now! To get your limbs in the best shape for the day, you want to be exercising five times a week, and there's no harm in performing additional bursts of exercises such as 20 press-ups and 30 squats every night before bed. These little extras take all of five minutes, but can make a huge difference.

One week before...
BRIDAL BEAUTY

A spray tan is best applied two days before the wedding, while semi-permanent eyelashes should be applied around five days before. A manicure and pedicure is the last thing you should do on the day before your wedding. Make sure your hands and cuticles are well moisturised that week, to help make them more pliable, and be prepared to allow the polish to dry for a good few hours before handling objects to prevent any unnecessary damage.

24 hours to go...
TRY TO RELAX!

Have a warm bath with bath salts to help reduce water retention, draw out toxins, neutralise your body's pH balance and help you relax before your big day. Now is not the time for a sentimental all-nighter with friends and family – you need to try to get a good night's sleep to avoid under-eye shadows, look well rested the in the morning and have the energy to enjoy every single moment.

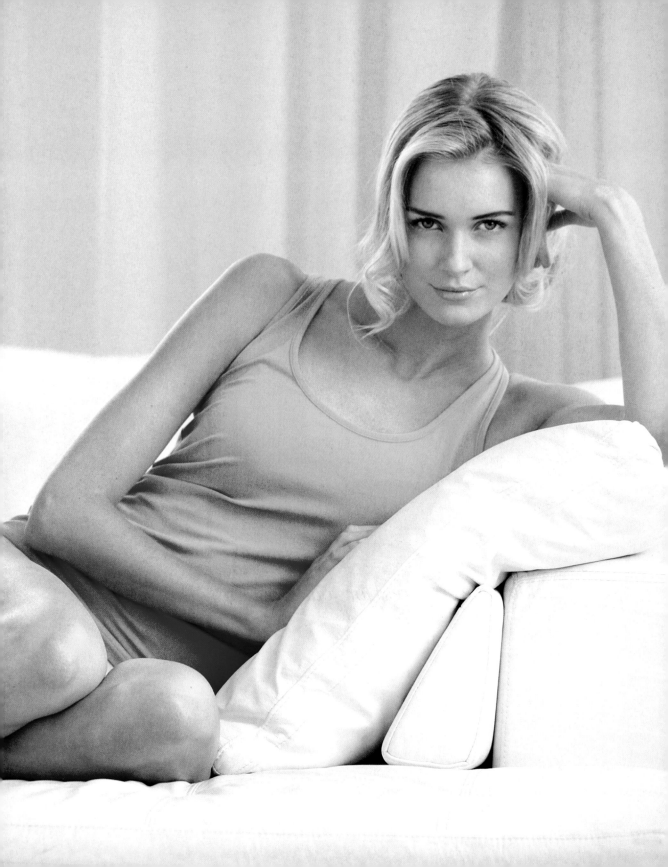

Body confidence

Ready to begin your transformation into a radiant, happy and beautiful bride? Looking and feeling great isn't just about losing weight and toning up. Beauty comes from within, so we're going to show you the techniques you need to feel confident, self-assured and gorgeous from the inside out. From perfecting your posture to finding the best dress for your shape, discover all you need to know to walk down the aisle in style!

A confident you

If you like who you are, you'll instantly look more beautiful, self-assured and happy - here's how to boost your self-belief

Every bride wants to look beautiful on her wedding day. But the secret is not about having the perfect body or wearing a size 8 wedding dress – it's about believing you are beautiful. When you feel confident, you exude happiness, contentment and beauty from within. Start working on accepting and believing in yourself now and in the run-up to your wedding, and you'll be able to look back on your wedding photos and see a joyful, radiant and happy bride looking right back at you. Read on to discover helpful tips and exercises that will get your confidence levels soaring and help you to enjoy being the centre of attention on your special day.

BE HONEST

To start building your inner confidence, you need to work on accepting yourself. Stand in front of a full-length mirror (you don't have to be naked, but it helps) and take a good look. For every 'flaw' you pick on, find two things you like about yourself. For example, you might hate your wobbly tum, but realise you have fantastic, shapely legs and beautiful skin.

This is not always an easy exercise to do, but once you start acknowledging all the great things about your physical appearance and playing down the not-so-great things, you can start to feel more positive about yourself. If there are any bits of your body that you really dislike, remember that you are going to improve them with a healthier lifestyle, which will enhance your best bits even more!

'Learn how to take a compliment - you're going to be receiving loads on your big day'

GET FEEDBACK

Sit down with your partner and (deep breath) ask him to tell you all the reasons why he loves you so much. When he gives his answers, try not to cringe – you're going to need to learn how to receive a compliment, because you'll be receiving loads on your big day! Make sure you listen and, most importantly,

accept what he tells you. While you might think you have a disproportionately large, cellulite-ridden bottom that's in desperate need of toning up, you might be surprised to learn that he views your derrière as one of your best assets. Realise that what you perceive as flaws could actually be someone else's favourite thing about you, and that goes for personality traits, too. While you're at it, why not ask your friends for their feedback as well – it will all help you to realise just how lovable you truly are.

DO IT FOR THE RIGHT REASONS

For many women, the simple act of getting engaged prompts them to want to lose weight – even if they're a healthy size already. But let's be crystal clear on something: your partner has asked you to marry him because he wants and accepts you just as you are. If you decide you really do want to slim down for your wedding, make sure you do it for yourself and no one else. Try not to feel under pressure from friends, family or society's expectations to lose weight and look perfect – you'll only end up making yourself miserable. Remember, being thin won't make you happy. Take a ❯❯

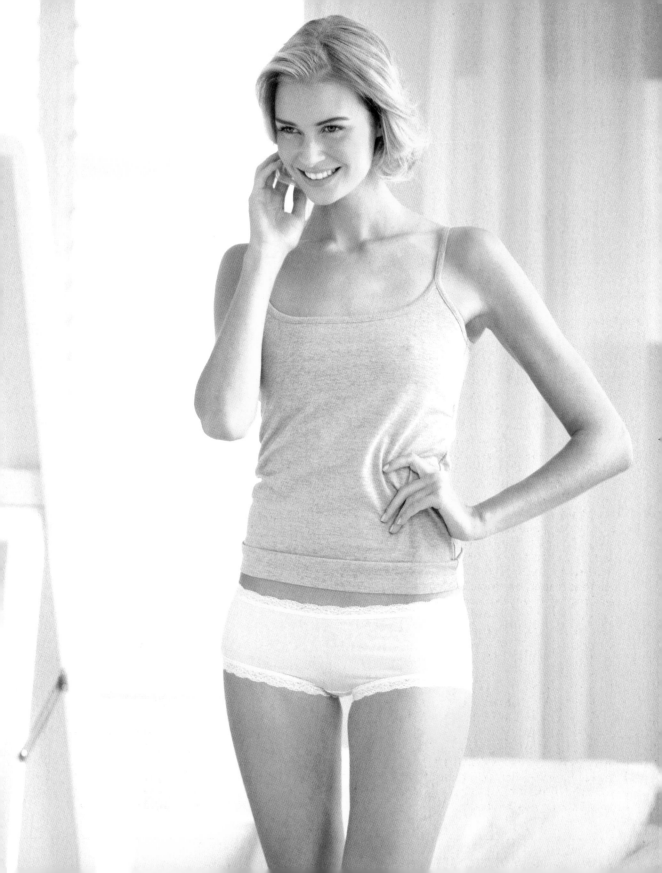

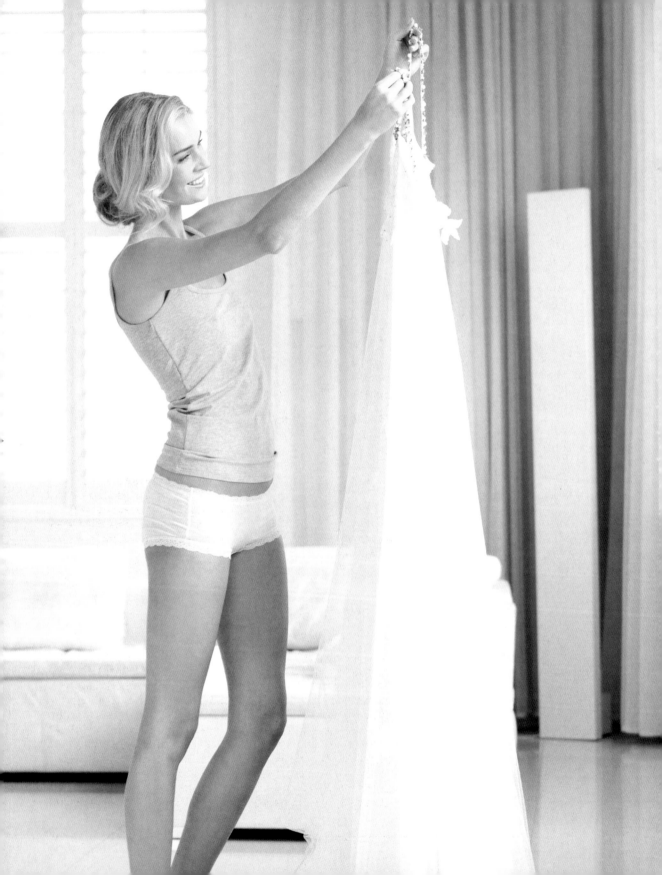

good look inside yourself and start to measure who you are with positive thoughts instead of pounds and inches. It might just be the greatest engagement gift you can give yourself.

BE REALISTIC
Every bride has a picture in her head of how she wants to look walking down the aisle, and this can be a powerful

> *'Measure who you are with positive thoughts instead of pounds and inches'*

motivator to help you to stay on track and reach your goals. But make sure this image is realistic and achievable for you. Trying to replicate the body of your favourite celebrity could cause you no end of stress. You need to accept now that there are some things you'll never be able to change about your figure – no matter how hard you diet and exercise – such as your height and basic bone structure. Instead, aim to make the most of what you have and look the healthiest you possibly can. You should look and feel happy because it's meant to be the happiest day of your life, not be miserable and stressed-out because you didn't end up looking like Cheryl Cole or Kelly Brook.

BE POSITIVE
Remember, you are in charge of your body, and it's up to you whether or not

you'll look your best. The majority of our favourite A-list celebs look fabulous because they train hard, lead healthy lifestyles and devote time to their beauty regimes – their great looks aren't always down to luck and good genetics. Losing weight and toning up can be as easy or as difficult as you want to make it. If you regard the changes you're going to make as positive, the greater your chance of success. For instance, when switching to a healthier diet, focus on all the delicious, fresh foods you're eating, rather than the things you think you're depriving yourself of. The same goes for exercise: concentrate on how much stronger, fitter and more energetic you are, instead of feeling deprived about missing an episode of your favourite TV programme while working out.

CHANGE YOUR BELIEFS
Your mind can be a powerful ally in helping you to achieve your goals, but only if you know how to use it properly. Your thoughts and feelings can either

drive you forward or hold you back. It's important that you realise your thoughts control your feelings; your feelings determine your actions; and your actions influence your behaviour. If you hold a negative thought about yourself, chances are it could sabotage your efforts at success. For example, if you've failed to lose weight in the past, you may think you'll never succeed at it, or if you believe that you are 'naturally overweight', these thoughts will affect your behaviour, making it more likely you'll fall at the first sign of temptation and skip a workout or eat something unhealthy. It's like you're giving yourself a ready-made excuse to fail before you even really try! The answer is to change what you think and believe about yourself. Repeat positive mantras to yourself on a daily basis, such as 'I can lose weight' or 'I can be naturally slim', and constantly visualise how great you will look and feel when you reach your goal and are able to enjoy the increased energy and confidence that will bring.

VISUALISE YOUR GOALS
Try this mental technique to enhance you chance of success

Athletes use visualisation to improve their performance, but you don't have to be a gold medallist to tap into the strength of this powerful technique. Because your mind doesn't know the difference between what is real and what is imagined, creating a visual image of how you want to look on your wedding day can help your subconscious encode this picture just as if it actually happened. It will focus your mind on your goal and help you intuitively move in the direction you want. Give visualisation a go by

sitting or lying down comfortably, then closing your eyes and taking some deep, relaxing breaths. Picture yourself walking down the aisle in your wedding dress. See yourself moving with confidence, and visualise every detail, from the glow of your skin to how it feels to be your perfect weight. Notice how this image makes you feel. Continue for five minutes (or longer if you prefer) and gently open your eyes. Do this on a daily basis, perhaps first thing in the morning or last thing at night, and you'll soon be on your way to making your visualisation a reality.

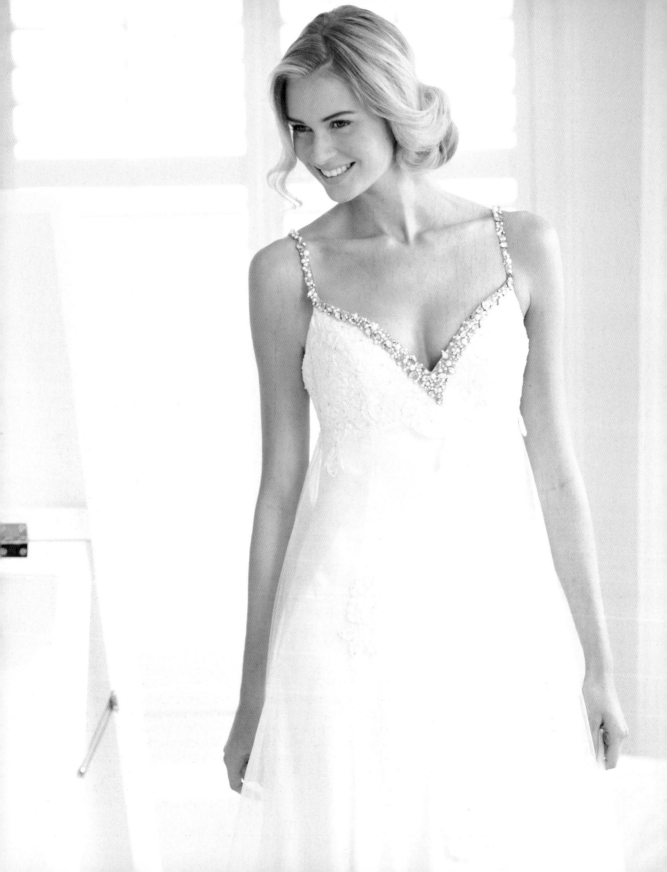

Find your DREAM DRESS

It will be a day you remember forever – and the photos will be seen for generations – here's how to pick the right outfit!

Shopping for a wedding dress is possibly the most exciting part of planning your wedding. And when you eventually find 'the one', it can make your impending nuptials suddenly seem that much more real (cue champagne-fuelled tears all round!).

But the fact is, finding the perfect dress can be a stressful and frustrating business. There's so much to consider, from different fabrics and styles to appropriate underwear and accessories. While it's fun to try on wedding dresses with your mum, sisters, aunties, grandmas and friends, don't make a firm decision about your dress without having someone who knows you inside out – and whose judgement you trust implicitly. Just because you've fantasised about having a certain style dress since you were a little girl, doesn't mean it will work for your figure. The wrong dress could add years and pounds onto you, leaving you feeling frumpy rather than fantastic on your big day.

So before you splash out, read our guide to learn which styles are best for your shape, and discover which areas of your body might require a little extra toning to do full justice to your dress. Happy shopping!

THE BEST DRESS FOR YOUR SHAPE

The right dress can accentuate your best bits and draw the eye away from parts you're not happy with. Read on to find out your body type.

HOURGLASS SHAPE

Your top and bottom halves are perfectly balanced, and you have a defined waist. In theory, your well-proportioned figure can carry off any style, including A-line and dropped-waist designs, but you're best suited to dresses that accentuate your waist, showing off your best asset. Trumpet and mermaid-style dresses that flare out at the mid-thigh or knees will cling to your curves in all the right places, while two-piece gowns can emphasise your waist further.

DO try dresses with built-in corsets to pull your waist in even more, and opt for sweetheart and bodice necklines if you want to accentuate your bust. Stick to simple, clean silhouettes.

DON'T swamp your curves in empire-line dresses or ball gowns. As your hips and chest are already balanced, you should also avoid having any extra detailing at these areas, so you don't appear top- or bottom-heavy.

TRIANGLE SHAPE

You are wider at the top of your body, with hips that are narrower than your shoulders. To balance your figure, you should look for dresses with full skirts that start from the waist, such as ball-gown and A-line styles. Empire line, sheath, trumpet and mermaid designs will only highlight your lack of hips. V-neck and scooped necklines work well to cover up wider shoulders, as do sleeves and wide shoulder straps.

'The wrong dress can add years and pounds onto you, leaving you feeling frumpy'

DO look at options with unusual or interesting details, such as embroidery, ruffles and bows around the middle and bottom of your dress, as this will force the eye downwards.

DON'T go for anything that draws attention to your shoulders, such as puffed sleeves, halter necks and off-the-shoulder dresses. Steer clear ≫

of embroidery and embellishment at the chest area if you want to avoid drawing attention to an ample bosom.

APPLE SHAPE

You have full breasts, a bit of a tummy and a rounder bottom and hips. More voluptuous than most, the best style for you is an empire-line dress that will de-emphasis your middle and give you a

> *'Don't add extra inches to your figure with details such as bows and ruching'*

leaner look. Corseted or basque styles can draw attention to your torso and, rather than hold you in, could create unattractive 'spillage' around your back, bust and under-arms.

DO opt for designs with straps if you need extra support, but avoid thin spaghetti straps that can cut into your shoulders. Invest in a well-fitting, supportive bra and wear 'magic' underwear to smooth out lumps and bumps.

DON'T add extra inches to your figure with unnecessary details such as bows, ruching and ruffles – stick to clean and simple lines to streamline your figure.

PEAR SHAPE

You are smaller on top than the bottom, with narrow shoulders, a small bust and generous hips and thighs. Ball-gown and A-line styles are perfect, as they disguise your lower half and put the focus on your torso and bust, emphasising your best bits. Floaty empire-line dresses can also work because they skim over your body from beneath your bust and highlight the smallest part of your body. Look for styles with lots of detail, such as ruching and embellishment at the chest.

DO go for halter necks, cap sleeves and strappy styles, to make the most of your petite shoulders. Pretty capes and bolero jackets also draw the eye upwards.

DON'T try trumpet and mermaid styles which will only draw attention towards your bottom and thighs. Sheath-type dresses can also cling to your more generously proportioned lower half, so don't be tempted by these styles.

CELERY SHAPE

Naturally slim, your figure tends to be straight-up-and-down, and you don't

have much of a waist. Your shape benefits from corset styles that will help to pull you in and create curves. When it comes to embellishment, you're one of the lucky few that can afford to go to town with ruffles, gatherings, big bows and tiers galore, especially around the bust and hip areas.

DO avoid empire-line dresses that will only emphasise your straight-up-and-down shape. But don't rule out sheath dresses – your slim figure lends itself to this close-fitting style as long as it's well cut, and isn't just shapeless.

DON'T skimp on underwear. Just because your boobs don't need support and you don't have any 'fat' areas, it doesn't mean your silhouette won't benefit from some figure-enhancing boosting and smoothing shapewear.

PETITE BRIDES (5' 1" and under)
Most silhouettes will flatter you, but ball gowns, mermaid and trumpet dresses can overwhelm your frame. Simple sheath and A-line dresses are best.

TALL BRIDES (5' 9" and above)
You can carry off almost any style, particularly mermaid and A-line dresses, but stay away from empire-line styles which can look tent-like.

The right lingerie

Finding the right foundation garments is essential to do justice to your figure and dress. Here are the things you need to consider when buying your bridal lingerie.

◆ **COMFORT:** Your wedding day is going to be a very long one – full of sitting for extended periods, eating, drinking, dancing and posing for photos – so don't sacrifice comfort for looks.

◆ **FIT:** if you're trying to lose weight, by all means find the designs you like in advance, but don't purchase your underwear until the week before your wedding, otherwise you could end up with gaping bra cups and baggy knickers. A good fit is also crucial for good support. Get professionally fitted so you buy the right size.

◆ **LOOKS:** By day, no one will see your underwear, but what about when it comes to stripping off in front of your new husband later that night? If you need functional shapewear to go under you dress, perhaps you should invest in a second set of sexier lingerie for bedtime.

Alternatively, look for specific bridal shapewear designed to smooth lumps and bumps, *and* look attractive. We recommend the new bridal collection from Body Wrap Bride (shapewear. co.uk), available in White or Ivory, with lace panelling for a more feminine look.

◆ **UNDER COVER?** The last thing you need on your wedding day is to see your underwear peeping out from your dress, so make sure you try everything on together to double check. A strapless, multi-way bra might be useful for dresses with low backs or halter necks. Watch out for any VPL under sheath dresses, too.

TONE UP FOR YOUR DRESS

Fitted and strapless designs mean you may not be able to hide figure flaws under yards of taffeta. Once you've established which style will compliment your shape, decide which areas you need to tone up before your dress fittings.

BALL GOWN
Skip lower-body moves and focus on getting sleek, sexy, sculpted arms and shoulders.

EMPIRE LINE
Sculpt the parts of your body that will be on show – arms, shoulders, chest and back.

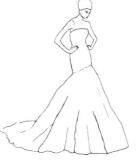

TRUMPET
Skimming your bottom and hips, this style needs a well-toned rear and sleek thighs.

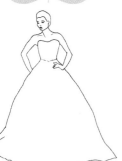

MERMAID
Ultra-snug, you'll need to whittle your waist, tone your thighs and lift your bum for this style.

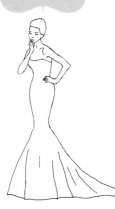

SHEATH
Without a built-in corset, a strong core is key. Also tone up your hips and outer thighs.

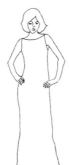

A-LINE
A-line styles give curvier waists a svelte look, but work better with flat, toned abs.

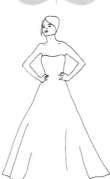

PICTURE PERFECT

Are you ready for your close-up? Learn how to strike a pose with these simple tips so you feel confident when all eyes (and cameras) are on you.

DO A TURN When standing, angle your body to 45° to create a slimmer profile. Avoid posing 'front-on', as this offers your widest silhouette to the camera. Tuck your hips under to conceal a larger bottom.

BE UPSTANDING Stand tall and upright, and keep your shoulders pulled back and tummy in to look your best from any angle. The same applies for sitting – no slouching!

EYE OPENER To avoid looking sleepy in every shot, try opening your eyes as wide as you can a few seconds before a picture is taken. And use eye drops to make your eyes glisten.

CALL TO ARMS Don't press your arms to your body – try holding them gently away from your torso so you can see the lines of your body. Also, to make them look more toned, slightly flex your arms.

DOUBLE TROUBLE If you're worried about a double chin, ask the photographer to hold the camera slightly above eye level and point the lens down when doing close-ups.

GET HIGH Always wear high heels (even if they can't be seen under your dress), as this will help give you a more feminine stance and the illusion of height.

DON'T HOLD BACK With all the posing you have to do, it can be easy to forget to enjoy the moment. Have fun, relax and show true emotion. You can always edit your photos later.

LAUGH OUT LOUD For a more natural smile, giggle when the photographer starts snapping (or ask someone to tell a joke).

Posture
PERFECT

Not only will it help you look slimmer, perfect poise can reduce fatigue and lower stress - just what you need on your big day

You've got the dress, the shoes, the lingerie, the veil and a fabulous bridal bouquet. Now there's only one other essential accessory – perfect posture.

Standing tall will make you look instantly slimmer, as well as give you the elegance and poise you need to glide down the aisle with grace. Unfortunately, many of us have poor posture as a result of sitting (read slouching) at a desk for long periods of time, standing poorly and leading inactive lifestyles. But the good news is that, with a little effort, you can strengthen your core, stretch out tight muscles and break bad postural habits. Follow our advice to realign your body and radiate confidence.

CHECK YOUR STANCE

Good alignment allows the joints in your body to be in a neutral position (not forced too far in one direction, or restricted in any way that can cause an imbalance), but your own posture may be very different. To determine your natural stance, put on some tight-fitting clothes and stand in a relaxed position in bare feet. Ask a friend to take photos of you front-on and sideways, to identify your posture trouble zones. Record the date on the photograph for reference.

WRITE A CHECKLIST

First, examine the picture – what do you see? When standing, your ears should be aligned over your shoulders, your shoulders above your hips, and your hips above your knees and toes. Your shoulders should be drawn back and down (not to be confused with sticking out your chest), your spine lengthened and your pelvis in a neutral position, not tilting forward or backward. Notice if you naturally slouch, or stand with your weight on one foot or with your pelvis tilted forward or back. Then, in front of a mirror, try to reposition your body to stand in good posture. Notice how this feels and what muscles you have to recruit to achieve it. Draw up a mental checklist of what you need to adjust and engage for ideal posture and, from now on, try to employ these corrections when you stand, sit and walk. Retraining your posture takes time, especially if you've developed bad habits. Try setting an alarm on your phone or computer at work every 30 or 60 minutes. When it goes off, readjust your posture until standing well becomes second nature.

ACTIVATE YOUR ABS

Rather than letting everything hang out, keep your core pulled in as you move about in everyday life. As well as helping to support your back and prevent injury, you'll end up with a flatter, more toned stomach, and will feel taller and slimmer, too. To find the right level, pull your abs in as much as you can (100 per cent). Relax, then pull them in to around 50 per cent. Relax again and, finally, draw your abs in to around 30 per cent – this is the level they should be held in all the time as you sit, stand and move around. Just remember to keep your shoulders relaxed, and breathe normally.

STRETCH REGULARLY

Regular stretching keeps muscles long and loose, and can help realign your body, too. As well as stretching out after your workouts, try doing some dedicated stretching sessions (after warming up thoroughly) to work on particularly tight areas of your body. Yoga and Pilates also help to elongate your body and keep you flexible. Sitting all day can lead to tight chest, abs and thigh muscles, and can eventually shorten the front of your body and pull you forwards, so stretch these areas regularly if you have a desk job.

CLOTHING Vest, £9 (pineapple.uk.com); Knickers, £4.95 (uniqlo.com)

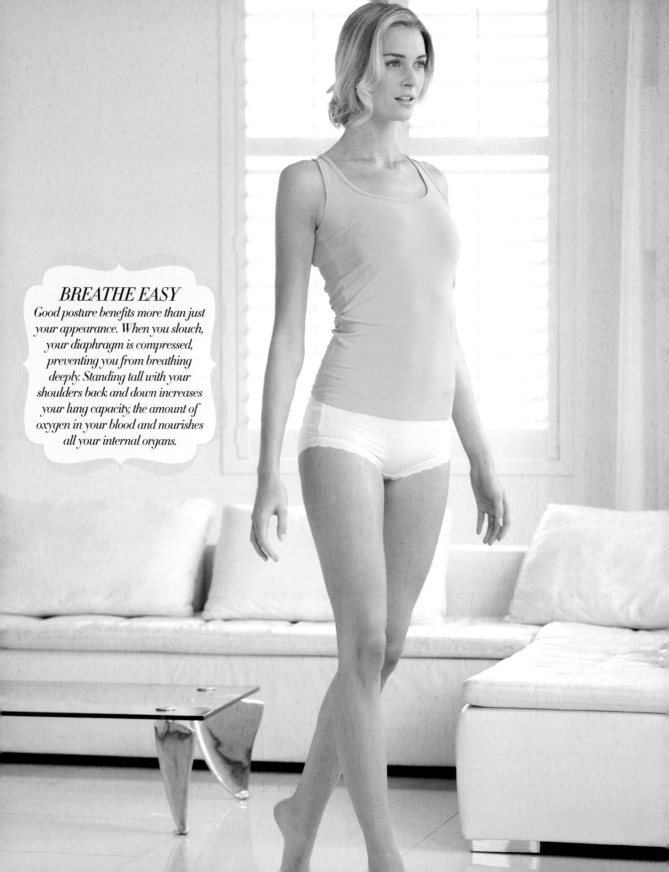

BREATHE EASY

Good posture benefits more than just your appearance. When you slouch, your diaphragm is compressed, preventing you from breathing deeply. Standing tall with your shoulders back and down increases your lung capacity, the amount of oxygen in your blood and nourishes all your internal organs.

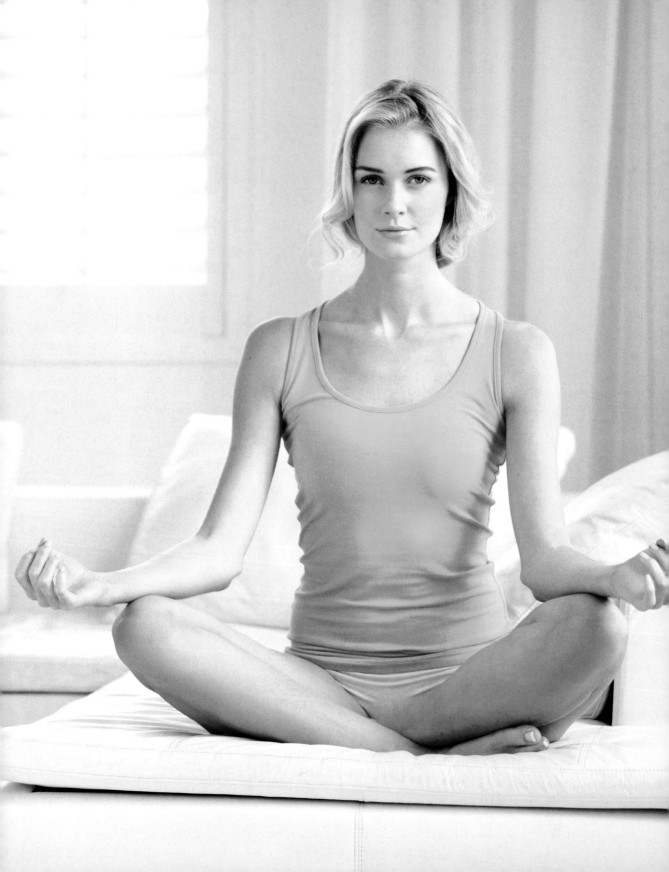

Beat STRESS

Planning a wedding takes time, energy and occasionally patience!
Sail through those tricky moments with our guide to keeping calm

The average bride-to-be makes a whopping 177 wedding-related decisions during her engagement, according to research. With so much on your mind, it's no wonder you can end up feeling a little frazzled. So try some of these stress-busting solutions to you help stay sane – and keep your inner Bridezilla at bay.

1 SET THE DATE

Deciding when to hold your wedding isn't as easy as you might think, and you may want to include both families in the conversation, especially if they don't live locally. Venues tend to get booked 12-18 months in advance, so you'll want to get this sorted as soon as possible. Other things you need to consider include: work schedules – select a time of the year when your work lives are less demanding and you'll be able take time off guilt-free; honeymoon – consider what type you want and whether weather conditions will be suitable at your chosen destination; other occasions – check if there are any big family celebrations or sporting events that could clash with your proposed date; your menstrual cycle – you want to look and feel your best on your big day, so avoid arranging your wedding when you're due on your period, especially if you suffer from PMS.

2 STAY ON BUDGET

Setting a budget for the ceremony and wedding reception is easy – it's sticking to it that's hard. Sit down with your partner to establish how much you have in savings (or not) and, if possible, talk with both sets of parents as early as possible to discuss how much they can contribute. Staying within your means can be tough, so it helps to determine a priority list for the ceremony and reception. Decide

{ *'Setting aside time to unwind is essential if you want to keep on top of things'* }

what really matters to you and which areas you can skimp on, so you and your partner have a clear idea from the start how your money is going to be spent. This should help avert potential arguments over spending later on.

3 SCHEDULE IN 'ME TIME'

Adding another 'must' on your to-do list might seem crazy now, but setting aside time to unwind is essential if you want to keep on top of

things. Try to allocate a couple of hours in your week for relaxation, put them in your diary and then make them non-negotiable. It doesn't matter whether you simply want a warm bath with some rejuvenating essential oils, a trip to the cinema or a natter with friends, just do whatever feels good for you. Another tip is to try and have one day of the week where you don't discuss or do anything related to your nuptials.

4 CUT OUT ALCOHOL

It's a sad fact that stress increases levels of the hormone cortisol in your body, which research shows increases the fat around your waist. But reaching for a glass of wine to help you relax can make the situation worse, as alcohol also raises cortisol levels (you have been warned!). Alcohol is also known to disturb sleep patterns, as your body has to work harder to remove toxins, which is why you often feel tired and lacking in energy the day after an evening of drinking.

5 BREATHE DEEPLY

Stress causes you to breathe rapidly, reducing the supply of oxygen to your brain and causing an increased heart rate, high blood pressure, tension and anxiety. However, breathing more deeply helps you take in extra oxygen and sends more blood » around your body. This lowers blood pressure and, in turn, tension and anxiety. Try a meditation class to learn how to control your breathing and get useful relaxation tips to use throughout the day. Find your nearest one at naturaltherapyforall.com.

6 REDUCE STIMULANTS

With so much to do, you might be relying on more caffeinated drinks than usual to get you through the day. Don't. It's likely you're already more anxious or nervous than normal, and caffeine and cigarettes – as stimulants and irritants to the nervous system – are only going to increase tension levels further.

7 SLEEP WELL

Make getting a good night's sleep a priority, to reduce stress, keep your mind sharp, and give you more energy. Stick to a regular routine, going to bed and getting up at roughly the same time every day to maintain your circadian rhythms (your body's internal clock), and aim to get at least seven hours a night. Try writing in a journal a few minutes before bed to unload the stressors that can cause insomnia and sleep disturbances. Avoid TV, computer and phone use an hour before going to bed (they can act as stimulants), and wear ear plugs and an eye mask, if necessary, to reduce light pollution and noisy sounds.

8 BE NATURAL

If your diet is lacking, try taking magnesium and zinc supplements to enhance your inner calm and improve your ability to cope with stress. Also try herbal remedies such as Bach Rescue Remedy (nelsonsnatural world.com) for stress relief on the go. Treat yourself to a monthly aromatherapy massage to soothe away stress, or try reflexology, acupuncture or homeopathy to help balance your system.

9 GET ACTIVE

Different forms of exercise can help beat stress in different ways. Cardiovascular exercise releases endorphins – your body's natural feel-good hormones which 'switch off' stress-causing adrenaline – and elevates your heart beat to increase the amount of blood and oxygen delivered to your muscles. This relieves muscular tension and makes you feel less constricted and able to breathe more easily. Mind-body exercise such as yoga, Pilates or t'ai chi helps to remove the physical and mental stressors of day-to-day life, and

{ *'Writing in a journal before bed can help unload stressors'* }

rebalances the physical efforts of strength and endurance exercise. Research shows that exercising outdoors – particularly in green, leafy areas – can also promote feelings of calm.

10 STAY FOCUSED

When things get stressful, and you face problems with the venue, caterers, photographer or family, step back and remember what your wedding day is really about – a celebration of love. Accept now that things won't always go according to plan and that you can't control everything, and you'll have a much more relaxed, fun time planning your wedding.

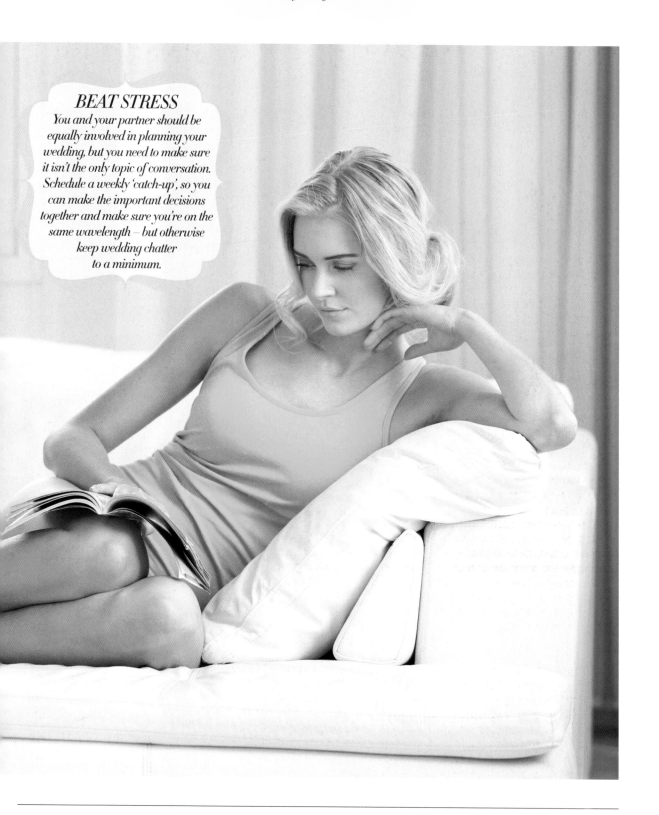

BEAT STRESS
You and your partner should be equally involved in planning your wedding, but you need to make sure it isn't the only topic of conversation. Schedule a weekly 'catch-up', so you can make the important decisions together and make sure you're on the same wavelength – but otherwise keep wedding chatter to a minimum.

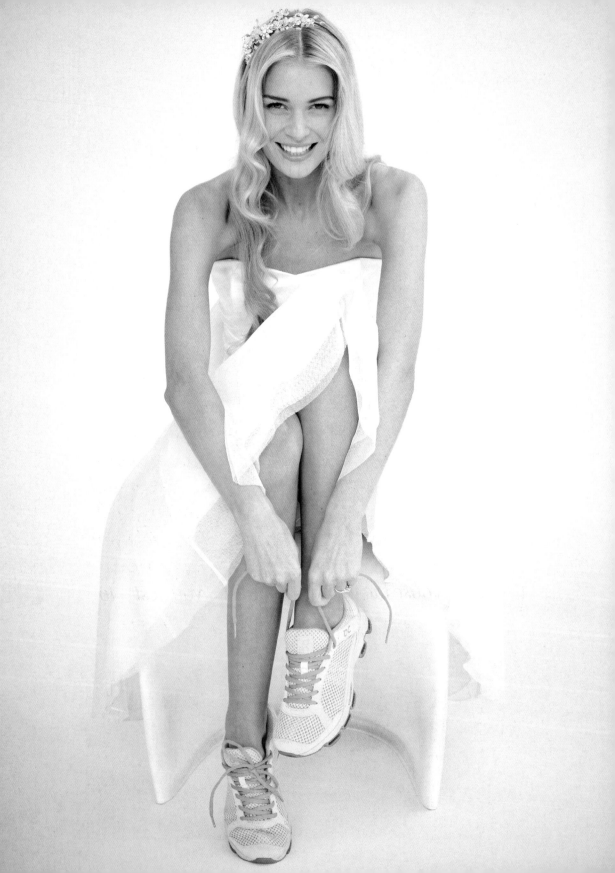

Get in shape

Now you know how to love yourself as much as your hubby-to-be does, it's time to discover the many reasons you should get fit – not just for your wedding day but for the rest of your life. Exercise not only makes you feel more energetic, healthier and happier; it can help you to look younger and enjoy a better sex life, too! In this chapter, you'll also find fitness and personality tests to help you determine your correct entry level into exercise and choose the workouts that suit you best – to make getting fit as fun and easy as possible.

Why get fit?

From being slim and toned for your wedding to protecting your health, here are all the amazing reasons why you should start exercising today!

Whether you're already working out or not, chances are you have your dream body in mind for your wedding. But trying to find time to exercise can seem stressful when you've still got all those invitations to send out, menus to choose and seating plans to arrange.

This is when it's good to remember that the benefits of a regular exercise regime will extend far beyond having bouquet-tossing-worthy biceps for your big day. Working out can also help save your sanity in the months leading up to the ceremony, and encourage you to develop a set of healthy fitness habits that you can maintain long after you exchange your vows, so you and your new husband can enjoy a long and happy life together.

THE HEALTH BENEFITS

Exercise offers a whole host of preventative and curative health benefits. It's been shown to reduce the risk of developing conditions ranging from heart disease, stroke and high blood pressure, to diabetes and osteoporosis, and can help keep your cholesterol levels healthy. You'll also be less prone to PMS, as well as the colds and other bugs that attack a weakened immune system.

THE MIND BENEFITS

Exercise triggers the release of feel-good chemicals called endorphins that can help combat stress, boost your mood

'Exercise can save your sanity in the months leading up to the wedding'

and lift depression to enhance your wellbeing. Research shows exercise can also help alleviate sleep problems and reduce cigarette cravings if you're trying to quit smoking. Additionally, working out can give you some well-deserved 'me' time (ideal for thinking though any problems you have), or the chance to socialise with friends and family.

THE BODY BENEFITS

As well as helping you tone your body, lose inches all over and reduce cellulite, exercise boosts your metabolism and maintains lean muscle mass, which prevents your body from storing excess fat. Additionally, as you lose weight, there will be less pressure on your joints and you'll move with more ease and energy, your posture will improve to help you stand taller and your limbs will become longer and leaner.

THE BEAUTY BENEFITS

It's official: exercise can slow the ageing process and help you look younger. By stimulating your circulation, it gives you a fantastic post-workout glow, nourishes your skin cells with oxygen and nutrients, and carries away waste products, cleansing your skin from within. Increased blood flow also stimulates your hair follicles, resulting in stronger hair that not only shines with health, but will grow quicker, too. Exercise can also help you sleep well at night – the key time your body secretes a growth hormone that helps repair and rebuild tissues, and plays a big part in maintaining skin-firming collagen. »

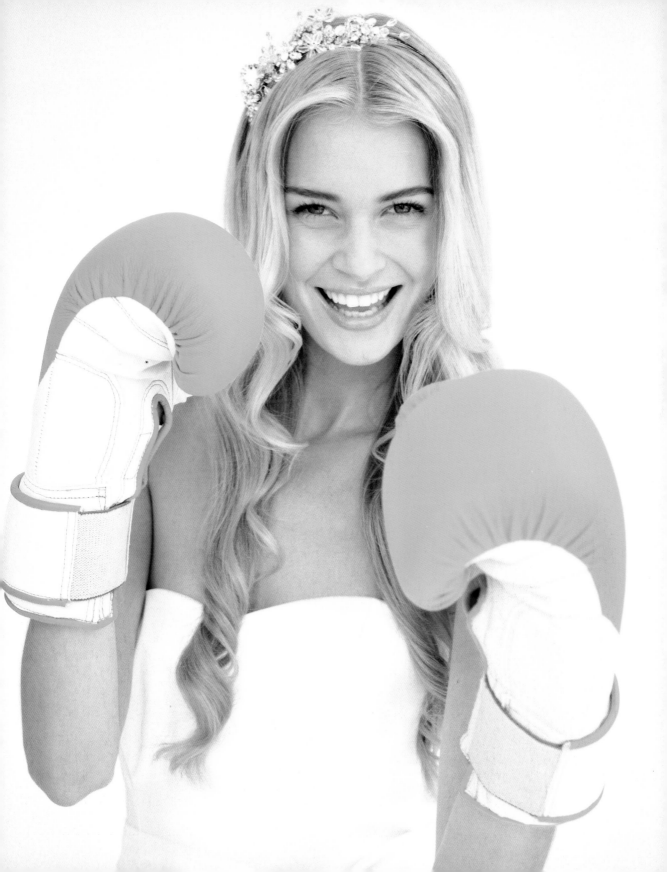

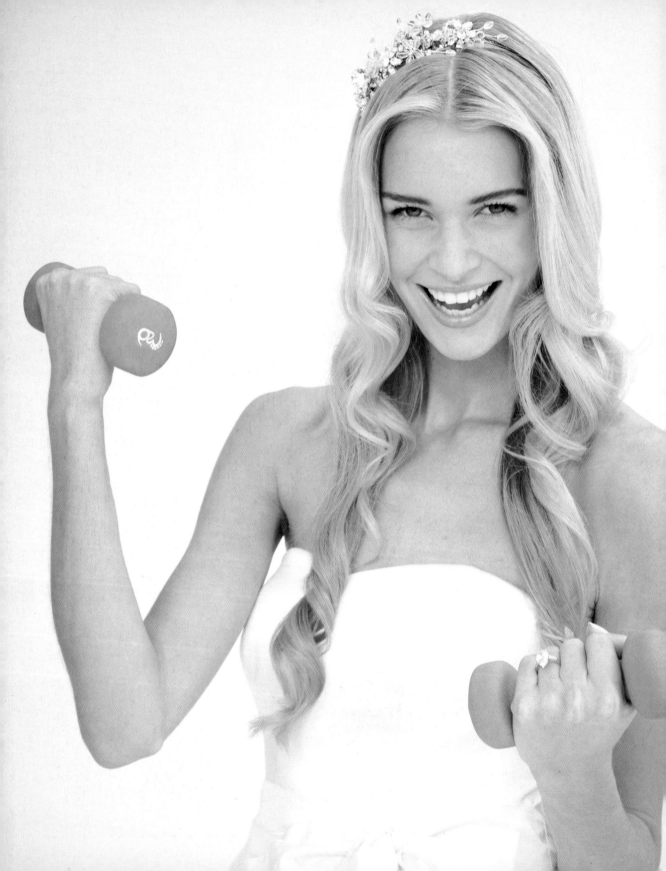

GET FIT NOW!

You don't need a gym membership or fancy equipment to start getting fitter – just get up and start moving!

Simply being more active will burn more calories than sitting still. Try to increase your daily moderate activity levels alongside doing the workouts in this book. For example, take the stairs instead of lifts and escalators, get off the tube or bus a stop earlier than usual and walk the rest of the way to your destination, go for a brisk walk in your lunch break or do some gardening or housework after work instead of flopping on the sofa. You'll soon turn your body into a calorie-burning machine.

One way to make sure you're being active enough is to wear a pedometer. You might be surprised how easy it is to miss the recommended 10,000 steps a day, especially if you have a job that keeps you desk-bound. Tracking your steps throughout the day makes it easier to keep tabs and factor in more walking if necessary. Pedometers cost around £20-£30, and good brands include Tanita (tanita.co.uk) and Omron (omron.co.uk). Alternatively, turn your smart phone into a pedometer with an app – try iStep for iPhone or Extra Pedometer for Android.

CHANGE YOUR ATTITUDE

To be your fittest and sexiest ever, it's not just your body that needs to change, but also your mind-set. If you see exercise as something to squeeze in around your job, friends and family, you'll always find excuses to avoid it. So make time for exercise by planning your workouts and putting them in your diary. Think of these sessions as if they are important business meetings you can't back out of, until fitness becomes a part of your lifestyle. Once you start seeing positive changes in your body and wellbeing, you won't want to miss your sessions.

Aim to maximise your training by staying as focused as possible, and ditch bad fitness habits, such as reading, watching TV or stopping to chat with friends while exercising. The more effort and concentration you put in, the better your results will be.

Don't judge your body solely on how it looks – enjoy the benefits you gain as you get stronger, fitter and more flexible. This will help you stick to your goals in the long term. For example, one week you might find you don't lose anything on the scales, but your strength or cardiovascular fitness may increase dramatically. This will help you lose more weight in the long term, as you'll able to train harder.

ESSENTIAL WORKOUT ADVICE

Make the most of your exercise sessions with these insider tips

ALWAYS SIP WATER before, during and after your workout to keep your body hydrated, and to replace lost fluids. Avoid eating big meals up to two hours before your training sessions.

WEAR A GOOD QUALITY, well-fitting sports bra when exercising to protect your breasts from any potential damage that bouncing can cause; try lessbounce.co.uk for a good selection.

WEAR TRAINERS that give you plenty of support during your workouts. Buy trainers at least half a size bigger than your regular shoe size, to allow your feet room to expand as they get hot.

CHOOSE CLOTHING that lets you move without restriction. If your budget allows, invest in gym gear with sweat-wicking properties to keep you dry and comfortable.

Fit for the bedroom

As well as giving you a stronger, more flexible body – plus oodles of energy, stamina and self-confidence – being fit also helps you have more intense orgasms. Get ready for mind-blowing sex with the following moves...

◆ The plié squats on p118 will tone your inner thighs, and indirectly tighten your vaginal walls and pelvic floor to enhance and intensify orgasms. Remember to stretch your inner thighs to maintain openness in the hips.

◆ Your glutes are rich with nerve endings, and you can increase orgasmic sensation by being able to maintain tension there. The low-as-you-can-go lunges on p115 mimic this tension as you squeeze your butt up and down.

◆ Good core stability equals stronger orgasms, particularly if you do exercises that target your lower abs, as these strengthen the pelvic muscles which contract during orgasm. Get toning with the bicycle criss-cross on p105.

◆ Sex-fit arms aren't just strong – they're adaptable, too. Try the full walking plank on p103; it will give you better balance and stability in your arms. You'll be springing into the 'naughty wheelbarrow' quicker than you can do a biceps curl.

◆ Having strong pelvic floor muscles boosts your arousal, provides more intensive orgasm contractions and feels great for your partner when you 'squeeze' him during intercourse. Locate your pelvic floor muscles by imagining you are stopping your pee mid-flow, without clenching your thighs or bottom. Then, flex these muscles 12 times, three times a day, in a pattern of two fast contractions then one held one. Eventually, try it during sex, and enjoy explosive results!

How fit ARE YOU?

Make sure you're ready to get in shape with these simple health and fitness tests

Following a regular exercise regime is incredibly beneficial for good health and wellbeing. But if you're new to exercise, recovering from an injury or have a niggling health problem, it's always best to have a quick health assessment before you start working out, to make sure you don't overdo it and cause further problems.

Read through the health checklist below, and if you answer 'yes' to any of the questions, see your doctor before exercising. Discuss your fitness plan with your GP to make sure your exercise is in step with your general health.

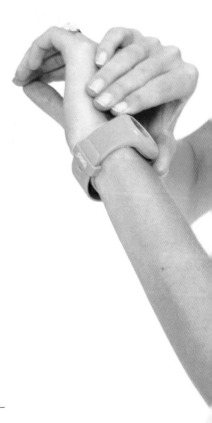

Your fitness MOT

◆ Have you been inactive for a year or more? Yes ☐ No ☐
◆ Have you ever been diagnosed with a heart condition or high blood pressure? Yes ☐ No ☐
◆ Do you smoke or are you a former smoker? Yes ☐ No ☐
◆ Do you have asthma or have you suffered from asthma? Yes ☐ No ☐
◆ Is there a history of premature heart problems in your immediate family (parent or sibling — under 55 in men, under 65 in women)? Yes ☐ No ☐
◆ Do you ever experience chest pain or dizziness during exercise? Yes ☐ No ☐
◆ Have you been diagnosed with a chronic bone or joint problem, such as arthritis or osteoporosis? Yes ☐ No ☐
◆ Are you diabetic? Yes ☐ No ☐
◆ Are you trying for a baby, pregnant or have you recently given birth? Yes ☐ No ☐
◆ Do you have a BMI (body mass index) of more than 26? Yes ☐ No ☐
◆ Have you been diagnosed with a chronic condition that may cause problems? Yes ☐ No ☐

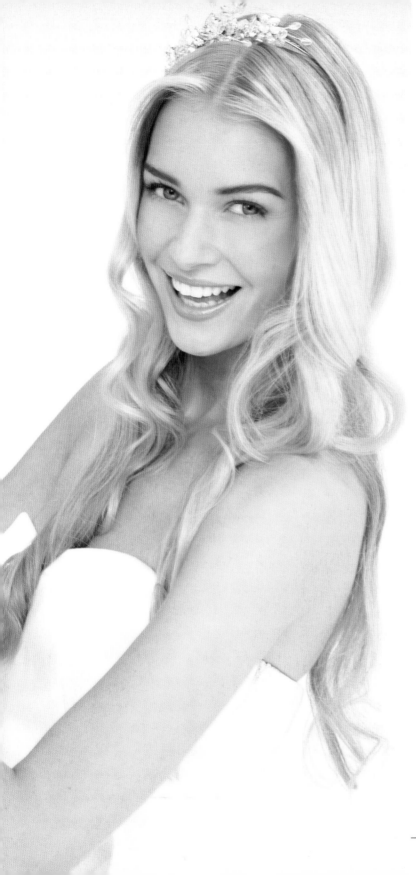

CHECK YOUR HEART RATE

Keeping tabs on your heart rate is a great way to check if you're getting a good workout. Your resting heart rate (RHR) is a good indicator of your general health, a normal rate for adults ranging from 60 to 100 beats a minute (bpm). Generally, a lower heart rate at rest suggests more efficient heart function and better cardiovascular fitness. For example, a well-trained athlete might have a normal resting heart rate closer to 40 beats a minute.

Find your pulse by placing two fingers on the inside of your wrist, neck or temple, or by using a heart rate monitor. The best time to take your resting heart rate is when you're lying down, having not exerted yourself.

Count your pulse for 15 seconds then multiply the number by four. This is your RHR. You'll be able to measure your improving fitness levels by timing how quickly it takes you to return to your resting heart rate after each workout. ≫

{ 'Your resting heart rate (RHR) is a good indicator of your general health' }

TEST YOUR FITNESS

Before you begin your new fitness regime, it's a good idea to establish your fitness levels in the areas of strength, cardio and flexibility. This will help you determine your correct level of entry into exercise, so you can train effectively and stay injury free. You'll also have invaluable benchmarks against which to measure your progress.

Complete the three tests below and record your results. Don't panic if they are lower than you'd like them to be – you'll soon improve. Retake the tests every four weeks and you'll be able to monitor exactly the fitness gains you are making, which will give your motivation a massive boost and help you keep on track.

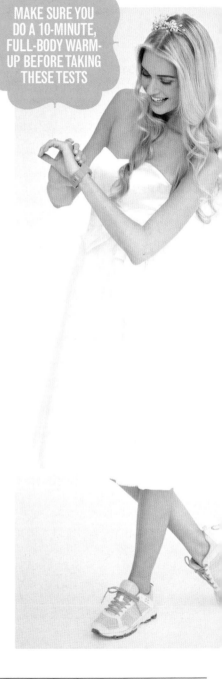

MAKE SURE YOU DO A 10-MINUTE, FULL-BODY WARM-UP BEFORE TAKING THESE TESTS

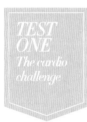

TEST ONE
The cardio challenge

WHAT TO DO Run 1.5 miles.
WHY DO IT? Measures cardiovascular fitness.
HOW TO DO IT Warm up by gently jogging for five minutes. Then, when your muscles are fully warmed up, time yourself running a distance of 1.5 miles. If you can't run for the whole distance, walk when necessary.

RESULTS

UNDER 30 YEARS OLD
14.01 mins or above below average
13.01-14.00 mins average
12.01-13.00 mins good
10.01-12.00 mins very good

30-34 YEARS OLD
14.31 mins or above below average
13.31-14.30 mins average
12.31-13.30 mins good
10.31-12.30 mins very good

35-39 YEARS OLD
15.01 mins or above below average
14.01-15.00 mins average
13.01-14.00 mins good
11.01-13.00 mins very good

40-44 YEARS OLD
15.31 mins or above below average
14.31-15.30 mins average
13.31-14.30 mins good
11.31-13.30 mins very good

45-49 YEARS OLD
16.01 mins or above below average
15.01-16.00 mins average
14.01-15.00 mins good
12.01-14.00 mins very good

50-54 YEARS OLD
17.06 mins or above below average
16.01-17.05 mins average
14.56-16.00 mins good
12.46-14.55 mins very good

55-60 YEARS OLD
18.11 mins or above below average
17.01-18.10 mins average
15.41-17.00 mins good
13.01-15.40 mins very good

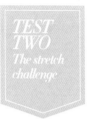

TEST TWO
The stretch challenge

WHAT TO DO The sit-and-reach stretch.
WHY DO IT? To assess flexibility.
HOW TO DO IT Sit on the floor (shoes off), with your feet 20cm apart against a bench. Keep your legs straight throughout. Bend at your hips, reach forward and mark the furthest point you can maintain for three seconds, in front of the bench (negative score) or on the bench (positive score).

RESULTS

-15cm or below very poor
-14 to -8cm poor
-7 to 0cm fair
+1 to +10cm average
+11 to +20cm good
+21 to +30cm excellent
(0cm is the point where your feet touch the bench.)

'If you do well in one area but not in others, focus more on these'

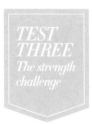

TEST THREE
The strength challenge

WHAT TO DO Sit-ups.
WHY DO IT? To measure abdominal strength.
HOW TO DO IT Lie on your back, feet under a sofa, knees bent and hands across your chest. With a flat back, raise your head, shoulders and torso until you're upright, then roll down to the starting position. Repeat for two minutes.

RESULTS

UNDER 30 YEARS OLD
0-39 below average
40-49 average
50-59 good
60-76 very good

30-34 YEARS OLD
0-37 below average
38-45 average
46-54 good
55-71 very good

35-39 YEARS OLD
0-31 below average
32-42 average
43-51 good
52-70 very good

40-44 YEARS OLD
0-26 below average
27-36 average
37-46 good
47-66 very good

45-49 YEARS OLD
0-24 below average
25-33 average
34-42 good
43-61 very good

50-54 YEARS OLD
0-22 below average
23-31 average
32-41 good
42-60 very good

55-60 YEARS OLD
0-20 below average
21-26 average
27-38 good
39-57 very good

Your entry level

◆ If you scored 'POOR' or 'BELOW AVERAGE', you're an exercise beginner. Start at week one of the six-week plan on page 123, and build up your fitness gradually. Your cardio sessions should consist of low-impact forms of exercise, such as walking, swimming or cycling until you're fit enough to progress onto running and high-impact aerobics. Don't worry if you can't manage all the repetitions in the main and target workouts. Just add another rep each time you train, and you'll soon get stronger and meet your targets.

◆ If you scored 'GOOD' or 'AVERAGE', you're an intermediate exerciser. You already have a good base level of fitness, but maybe you're not used to training very regularly. Start at week one of the six-week plan (page 123) unless you already train three to four times a week, in which case start in week two. Focus on good technique before going onto the progressive exercises. If you're fit enough, and already used to longer cardio sessions, add extra minutes onto the cardio sessions in the plan, and increase them accordingly, to make sure you're working hard enough.

◆ If you scored 'ABOVE AVERAGE' or 'VERY GOOD', you're an advanced exerciser. You have excellent fitness levels, but check if they are well balanced. You might be great at running, for example, but poorer in strength and flexibility. Focus on these for excellent overall fitness. If you already exercise four to five times a week, start in week four of the six-week plan on page 123 (never exercising more than five times a week). To continue to progress, increase the resistance and intensity of the exercises.

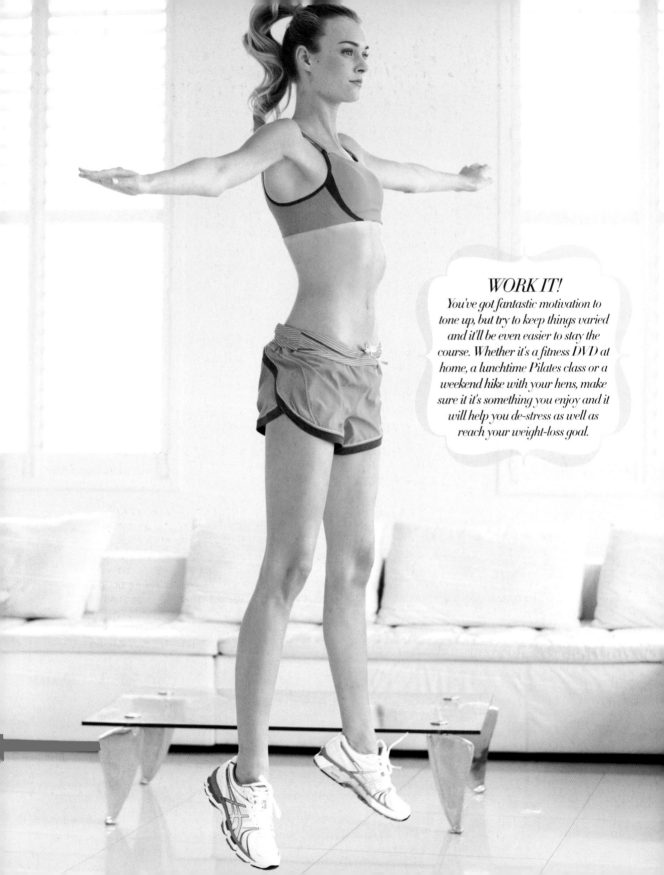

Find the best EXERCISE *for you*

If you don't enjoy your workouts, chances are you'll give up before too long. Here's how to match your training to your personality

N ow you know your fitness level, it's time to find out which types of exercise you should be doing – not just those that will help you reach your goals but, more importantly, those that will suit your lifestyle and personality. The key to sticking to any fitness regime is to do activities that you enjoy. Exercise should enhance your life and be pleasurable, and the minute you start doing activities because you feel you ought do them, rather than because you want to, you'll end up bored and demotivated, and might start finding reasons to avoid them.

Similarly, you need to choose workouts that fit your lifestyle. If you have a really stressful job, perhaps the last thing you should do is a hectic Spinning class – even if your goal is to burn tonnes of calories – because you'll still feel like you're working. But something like ashtanga yoga, for example, will give you a tough workout and calm you at the same time. Equally, if you're at home all day on your own or with children, and find yourself craving adult conversation, joining a running group or buddying up with friends for jogs will be much more rewarding for you than going out running on your own or doing a yoga DVD in your living room.

These days, we're spoilt for choice for workouts to try, so there's no excuse not to experiment and find the type that's perfect for you. Take our test on page 42 now to find out your fitness personality. Whether you're a self-motivator, a team player or a free spirit, discover which kind of fitness activities will keep you rushing back for more. »

CLOTHING: Jubralee crop top, £37 and momentum short, £30 (moving comfort), Gel-Kayano 18 trainers, £138 (asics.co.uk)

> *'Ashtanga yoga will give you a tough workout and calm you at the same time'*

TAKE THE TEST

When you were younger, your favourite way to be active was:
A A run around the block
B Making up dance routines with friends
C A walk through the woods, searching for treasures

The best time for you to work out is:
A Whenever I can; morning or night, weekdays or the weekend
B I'm fairly flexible – it doesn't really matter as long as I'm with my friends
C There isn't one time, my schedule changes all the time

The word that best describes you is:
A Driven
B Sociable
C Adventurous

The way you would most want to spend one active hour would be:
A With a personal trainer to make sure I'm getting the best workout
B Dancing the night away with friends or playing with teammates
C Trying a new activity, such as surfing or ultimate frisbee

When exercising, what motivates you to keep going is:
A Knowing I'm getting closer to my goals
B The thought of enjoying a post-workout drink with friends
C The fact that I know it will all be over soon

Your workout gear of choice would be:
A The latest, hi-tech, sweat-wicking designer kit
B A cute workout outfit I can show off to friends
C Just an old T-shirt and shorts – no one is looking at me anyway

When you feel stressed, you:
A Make a to-do list
B Call my nearest and dearest
C Meditate or take deep breaths

What it comes to workout music, you prefer:
A To put on my iPod and go
B Anything fun that gets me moving
C The sounds of nature

When playing board games, you most hope to:
A Win
B Have fun
C Learn something new

What's your fitness personality?

Mostly As? You're a... SELF MOTIVATOR

PERSONALITY: Organised and focused, you find it easy to stick to a programme, so you should have no problem finding the necessary discipline you need to follow our six-week shape-up plan (page 122). You're happy to exercise by yourself, but try doing one class or cardio session a week with a friend to make your training more fun. You tend to stick to the activities you feel comfortable with, so boredom can be a problem. Try a new workout once a month to shake things up, and mix up your cardio sessions with different activities.
WORKOUTS TO TRY: Kick-boxing; cycling; circuit training; swimming; Pilates; Body Pump; skipping; ballet; running; Spinning.

Mostly Bs? You're a... TEAM PLAYER

PERSONALITY: You favour group classes and team sports that let you catch up with friends. You thrive on camaraderie, but don't let your training fall by the wayside if a friend cancels on you. Choose activities you enjoy (not just the ones other people want to do), and avoid losing focus by getting too distracted with the latest gossip. Enlist a bridesmaid, family member or friend of a similar fitness level to follow our six-week plan with you (or at least to join you for the cardio sessions) to keep boredom at bay.
WORKOUTS TO TRY: Tennis; netball; aerobics; bootcamp-style classes; hockey; dancing; water aerobics; power walking; Zumba.

Mostly Cs? You're a... FREE SPIRIT

PERSONALITY: You love trying new things and dislike being tied down to a routine. You find it hard to stick to a workout programme, often exercising only when you feel like it. Random invites from friends suggesting a hike in the woods or a trip to the bowling alley get you moving. The key to your shape-up success is variety, so mix up locations, workouts and training buddies. Feed your love of freedom by exploring new places on your bike or doing something fun, like going to a roller disco.
WORKOUTS TO TRY Bollywood dancing; t'ai chi; hiking; Lindy hop; Nordic walking; golf; salsa; orienteering; mountain biking; yoga.

Play together, stay together!

Work out with your man for improved results, better communication and hotter sex...

Right now, you're focused on getting fit and looking amazing for your wedding day. This is great, but have you ever wondered whether your partner might be having exactly the same body hang-ups as you when it comes walking down the aisle with all eyes on the pair of you? Or perhaps your hubby-to-be is already super-fit but you've never spent any time exercising together before? Whether your man is a couch potato or buff beefcake, encouraging him to get involved in your new fitness regime could be one of the best things you do, not only to help you both get in better shape, but to bring you closer together than ever before.

TWICE AS GOOD

While exercising à deux might not seem the most romantic of pastimes, research shows couples who sweat it out side-by-side have more successful relationships, and even hotter sex lives – once they've wriggled out of their gym gear. The common bond you share through exercising together helps you inspire each other to achieve your goals. You'll also find your communication improves as you support each other through the training lows and celebrate the highs – something you don't get from watching a DVD together. It also stands to reason that if you've done something with your partner that makes you feel good about yourself (such as exercise), you're going to associate those positive feelings with your man, which can only be a good thing. If you're concerned your partner could end up being a hindrance to your fitness regime, think again. Research from Indiana University shows married couples who train together stand a 94 per cent chance of sticking with their training programmes, compared to the 43 per cent drop out rate of married people who exercise on their own, confirming that once you and your partner start exercising together, it's likely you'll be more committed to maintaining a regular workout regime that can continue long after you say your vows.

THE RULES OF THE GAME

Follow these easy tips to make your joint fitness activities even more successful

SET A GOAL Having a common goal – whether it's each losing half a stone or dropping a 'trouser' size – will help you share the ups and downs of the challenge. Enjoy the journey, not just the final result.

PLAN AHEAD Schedule dates in your diaries for joint exercise sessions and commit to them. Being organised can make the difference between trying a new activity after work or spending another night on the sofa.

EASY DOES IT Don't let a lack of fitness hold you back. Any activity – including a gentle walk or bowling – is better than none, and you'll still benefit from sharing the experience.

COMPROMISE Can't agree on a shared activity? Try going to the gym at the same time and just warm up and cool down together. You still get to talk to each other about your session plans and achievements, which can help you to understand each other better, and then come up with activities you would both enjoy.

FIND A BALANCE Maintaining a balance between exercising together and doing normal things, such as going out for a meal or socialising with friends, is important. Take time to relax with each other and don't get too obsessed with your exercise plans or weight-loss goals.

KEEP IT FAIR Find an activity that stays within both your fitness and ability levels, and that you both feel comfortable doing. Avoid pressuring each other to try activities that are too challenging, or make one of you feel embarrassed or uncomfortable.

Top couple workouts

Try some of these gender-neutral activities to get you in the mood to exercise together.

- ◆ SPINNING
- ◆ MARTIAL ARTS
- ◆ INDOOR CLIMBING
- ◆ CIRCUIT TRAINING
- ◆ WALKING
- ◆ RACKET SPORTS
- ◆ BOOTCAMP CLASSES
- ◆ SWIMMING

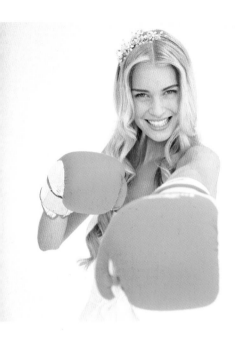

Why do CARDIO?

From boosting your circulation to increasing your metabolism, cardio exercise will shape you up in no time. Here's how

Cardio exercise, short for cardiovascular, is any movement that gets your heart rate up and increases circulation throughout your body. It provides a variety of health benefits, from strengthening your heart and circulatory system, to raising your metabolism and helping you burn off excess calories. There are many forms and methods of cardio exercise available to try – the key is choosing the right type for your fitness level, shape-up needs and personality.

MAKE CARDIO WORK FOR YOU

If you're just getting started, focus on finding an activity that you enjoy and that gets you moving. Then aim to gradually increase the number of times you do it and the length of your sessions – ideally, you should try to do three to five sessions a week, at a minimum of 30 minutes each.

If you're used to cardio, then it's time to shake up your sessions with different training states, including long slow duration (LSD) and interval training sessions (both of which feature in your six-week shape-up plan). Not only will these training techniques help boost your fitness and fat-burning levels even further, they will also help stave off boredom and keep things fun.

HOW HARD SHOULD YOU BE WORKING?

For cardio to be effective, you need to exercise at a level that raises your heart rate to your target zone. Research indicates that working within a target heart-rate zone of between 60 to 90 per

> *'You need to exercise at a level that raises your heart rate to your target zone'*

cent of your maximum heart rate is effective for most people, although if you're out of condition, working at 50 per cent may be enough to begin with. To work out your target zone levels, you must first establish your maximum heart rate. Do this by subtracting your age from 220 and then calculating 60 and 90 per cent of that number (the table opposite offers a rough guide).

Using a heart rate monitor can help you train within your target zone, but a cheaper alternative is to simply count your pulse beats, mid-exercise, for 15 seconds, then multiply that number by four to get the beats per minute. If the result is higher than the upper limit of your zone, you are working too hard and if it is lower, this indicates you can push yourself more.

LONG CARDIO EXPLAINED

Long slow duration (LSD) cardio involves working at a fairly low-intensity (around 60-80 per cent of your maximum heart rate) for an extended period of time,

'You can use interval training for any workout — at the gym, at home or outside'

usually for a minimum of 15 minutes and often up to an hour. LSD sessions improve cardiovascular fitness and lung capacity, so you will be able to push yourself harder in interval training (see right) and boost calorie burning.

You can choose any type of activity in keeping with your existing fitness levels (low-impact forms of cardio such as power walking and swimming are great for beginners, while more intense forms such as running and high-impact aerobics are ideal for intermediate and advanced exercisers). The important thing is to keep your heart rate steady throughout to improve your fitness. Each time you do an LSD session, try adding another three to five minutes on to the

time you managed previously, to further challenge your fitness levels.

INTERVAL TRAINING EXPLAINED

Interval training involves alternating spurts of high-intensity exercise (for instance, by increasing your speed, effort or incline for one minute) with moderate-intensity exercise (decreasing your speed, effort or incline for one minute, or until your heart rate has suitably reduced), and then repeating the process. This type of training is fantastic for strengthening your heart, because it gets you working at an intensity you wouldn't be able to maintain consistently during an LSD session.

Your muscles also develop more quickly, meaning you'll burn extra calories during your workout and for several hours afterwards when resting, because muscle burns more calories than fat. As interval training sessions are higher in intensity, they can be shorter than LSD sessions (a 10-minute burst can be as beneficial as a 30-minute LSD session), and you can incorporate this

Top workouts

Get active with one of these great forms of cardio:

- WALKING
- RUNNING
- SWIMMING
- DANCING
- CYCLING
- ROWING
- SPINNING
- BOXING
- ZUMBA
- AEROBIC CLASSES
- RACKET SPORTS
- NETBALL
- HOCKEY
- SKIPPING
- SKATING

type of training into any workout: on a treadmill or cross-trainer at the gym, with a flight of stairs at home or at work, or by using a hill outside.

To do interval training, perform a form of cardio that gets your heart rate up to around 70 per cent of its maximum level. Then, for a period of 30, 45, or 60 seconds (depending how long it takes you to get to around 85-90 per cent of your maximum heart rate), work at a high intensity by training harder or faster. Once you reach this level, immediately reduce your effort to allow your heart rate to slowly recover and return to around 70 per cent. You can repeat this sequence as many times as you want. For example, a 10-minute interval session could consist of a one-minute, high-intensity interval followed by a one-minute, low-intensity interval, multiplied by five.

Once you give interval training a go, not only will you see an improvement in your fitness levels, you'll also be lowering your risk of heart disease, type 2 diabetes, stroke and some cancers.

KNOW YOUR TRAINING ZONES

Use this table to calculate what heart rate zone to train at for maximum results.

AGE	AVERAGE MAXIMUM HEART RATE 100%	TARGET HEART RATE ZONE 60-90%
20-30	195	117-176 bpm*
31-40	185	111-167 bpm
41-50	175	105-156 bpm
51-60	165	99-149 bpm

(* beats per minute)

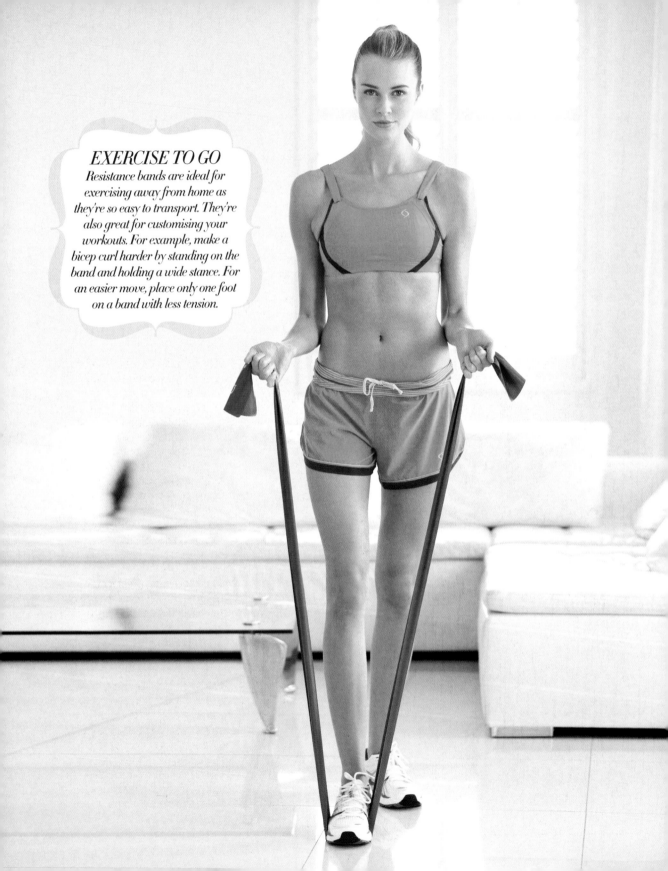

EXERCISE TO GO

Resistance bands are ideal for exercising away from home as they're so easy to transport. They're also great for customising your workouts. For example, make a bicep curl harder by standing on the band and holding a wide stance. For an easier move, place only one foot on a band with less tension.

Why do WEIGHTS?

Use resistance work to create a leaner, toned silhouette and look stunning in your wedding dress!

The benefits of weight training aren't just a strong, sexy and beautifully toned body. Lifting weights also helps to raise your metabolism and reduce body fat. What's more, it also lowers your blood pressure, reduces levels of bad cholesterol and cuts the risk of osteoporosis.

Unfortunately, many women (particularly brides-to-be) shun weight training, or don't use weights that are heavy enough, because they incorrectly assume they'll bulk up. In fact, using weights can help you achieve the lean and slender look you're after.

If you've been afraid to use weights for fear you'll get bigger rather than smaller, now's the time to put those doubts aside. The average women doesn't have enough testosterone to get 'big' – in fact, weight training actually has the opposite effect, because the more lean muscle you have, the higher your metabolism will be as your muscles require more calories to fuel them. For example, if you gain 5lbs of lean muscle, your daily burn will be hundreds of calories higher, meaning you can eat more calories than you might normally consume and still lose weight!

CHOOSE THE RIGHT WEIGHT FOR YOUR FITNESS LEVEL

To do the body-sculpting workouts in this book, you'll need a pair of dumbbells. Use light weights (1-2 kg) if you're new to weight training, medium weights (2-4 kg) if you're intermediate, and heavy weights (5-10 kg) if you're advanced. If you don't already have some, or you're a beginner, don't rush out immediately to buy a set. A cheap alternative is to use

'If you gain 5lbs of muscle, your daily burn will be hundreds of calories higher'

large water bottles filled with water (light resistance), sugar (medium resistance) or pebbles (heavy resistance). Just make sure they weigh an equal amount!

Bear in mind that some muscles are much stronger than others, so while a light weight might be perfect for biceps curls, it probably won't be heavy enough for lower-body exercises, such as squats

that incorporate weights. The weight you use to start with needs to be individual to your current strength, but as a general rule, your ideal 'free weight' (or dumbbell) should tire your muscles out after 12 to 15 repetitions of an exercise. When the 12th rep becomes easy, it's time to increase your weights by two or three pounds. Don't stay at the same weight when you know you can increase the resistance – make sure you always challenge yourself to achieve your perfect bridal body!

WEIGHT-TO-GO

While dumbbells are great for use in the home or at the gym, they're not exactly the easiest of things to transport around when you need to work out on-the-go. So why not give resistance bands a try? These long, stretchy bands are compact and super-lightweight, so you can stick one in your bag to take to the park for a spot of impromptu toning, or pack in your suitcase when you travel – perfect if you want to maintain your newly buff body on your honeymoon. Available in a range of resistances – colour coded for easy reference – you can also make them shorter or longer to create less or more tension.

Bridal bootcamps

*If you need some extra motivation,
a fitness retreat may be the answer*

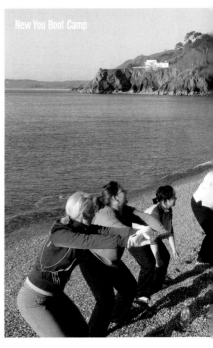

New You Boot Camp

Bootcamps promise fantastic weight-loss results and a drop in dress size in as little as seven days. But make no mistake, they are super-tough, even if you are über fit and used to training five days a week. For the best results, avoid using them as a last ditch attempt to fit into your dress a week or two before the big day. Good bootcamps advocate long-term solutions to healthy weight loss. They're not cheap either, so book one early to make use of everything you learn in the months leading up to your wedding.

THE CAMP

LOCATION **The Peak District; Galloway, Scotland; Andalucia, Spain**
CONTACT **thecamp.co.uk**

One of the oldest military bootcamps for women in the UK, The Camp has Special Forces trainers but a 'no shouting' policy in place, and you can expect to lose seven to nine pounds. There's time to reflect, assess your goals and experience the beauty of the great outdoors. You'll also gain life-long access to the online member's area, full of fitness tips and dietary advice.

NEW YOU BOOT CAMP

LOCATIONS **Suffolk; Somerset; Spain; Portugal; Austria; London (one-day groups)**
CONTACT **newyoubootcamp.com**

Choose from basic army-style camps – complete with bunk beds, a communal bathroom and washing your own dishes – to luxury retreats with all manner of pampering extras on offer. If you love the great outdoors, go for the latest Alps experience in Austria and torch calories with Nordic walking and mountain biking. All programmes aim to re-energise, inform and inspire you, and give support, tools and resources to make sure you continue to keep the weight off once you've returned home.

NO.1 BOOTCAMP

LOCATIONS **Kings Lynn, North Norfolk; Ibiza; Marbella**
CONTACT **no1bootcamp.com**

With a variety of locations close to the sea (some sunnier than others!), you can expect lots of gruelling beach runs and water workouts in addition to boxing, circuit training and hikes in the countryside. If you're short on time but want big results, opt for one of the shorter weekend-only or mid-week stays on offer, alongside the seven-, 14-, 21- and 28-day retreats. Mixing expert military-style training with sensible nutritional advice, plus optional beauty treatments including massages, facials, waxing, tanning and manicures, these camps are also popular with celebs who need to look red carpet-ready, pronto!

NUBEGINNINGS

LOCATIONS **North Devon; Loire Valley, France**
CONTACT **nubeginnings.co.uk**

It may be pricey, but you can expect to lose around 10lbs during a week's stay at Nubeginnings, while enjoying organic, locally-sourced food, luxury accommodation with Rhodes to Heaven and Elemis bath products, fitness assessment, three full-body deep-tissue massages to soothe aches and pains and use of the sauna. Also included are two hypnotherapy sessions that promise to get to the heart of emotional eating and an NLP (neuro-linguistic programming) goal-setting workshop.

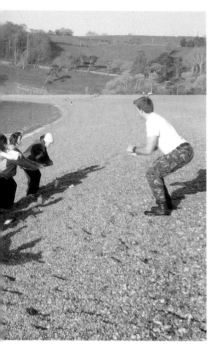

Bootcamp survival guide

Use these tips to get the most from your bootcamp experience.

◆ Make sure you're doing the bootcamp for you, not anyone else, and approach it with a positive mind-set.
◆ Detox your body before you go, ensure you're well hydrated before you start – drink herbal teas, cut out caffeine and alcohol and eat more raw fruit and veg.
◆ Get plenty of sleep to boost your energy.
◆ Take layers of clothes to help regulate your temperature, and wear gloves that cover your wrists. Treat yourself to some new kit and invest in a good quality pair of trainers fitted by a professional.
◆ Pack a mini first-aid kit, including pain killers, blister plasters and muscle rubs to soothe minor aches and pains. Take Epsom salts with you to bathe in at the end of the day to help your muscles recover.

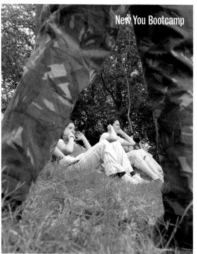

New You Bootcamp

BRIDESMAID BOOTCAMPS

It's likely it's not just you who's feeling the pressure to look great on your wedding day – your bridesmaids are probably feeling it too!

If this is the case, why not rope them into your fitness regime? You'll all benefit from the support you give each other, and have a load of fun and giggles at the same time. If you can't all afford to go on a residential bootcamp, try a one-day experience at one of the retreats above, or find a personal trainer in your area who could help cater for your needs (find yours at exerciseregister.co.uk). Alternatively, British Military Fitness (britmilfit.com) runs hundreds of army-style outdoor fitness group sessions all over the UK, and you can even try a session for free to see if it's something that suits you and your friends.

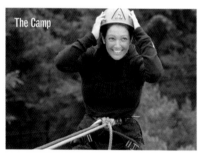

The Camp

GI JANE BOOTCAMP

LOCATION Sittingborne, Kent
CONTACT gijanebootcamp.co.uk

This women-only camp claims to have the best ratio of instructors to clients of any bootcamp in the UK. The team of expert health coaches and councillors offers support to help you through the challenging programme of boxing, running, skipping, cycling, core training and water activities, plus volleyball, netball, obstacle courses and war games. The camp believes in nourishing you fully for all the activities, so no food groups are excluded – including carbs!

KICK-START BOOTCAMP

LOCATION Newark, Nottinghamshire
CONTACT kick-startbootcamp.co.uk

Expect assault courses and team-building exercises galore on this military-style bootcamp, which promises to help you drop a dress size and tone up. If you're time-poor, try the four-day course for a motivational boost and to lose some pounds as well. If you're not sure you'd like a bootcamp, there are one-day taster courses available. Or try an adventure weekend abroad, where you and your husband-to-be can have fun together while losing weight to boot.

'If you can't afford a residential camp, try a one-day experience'

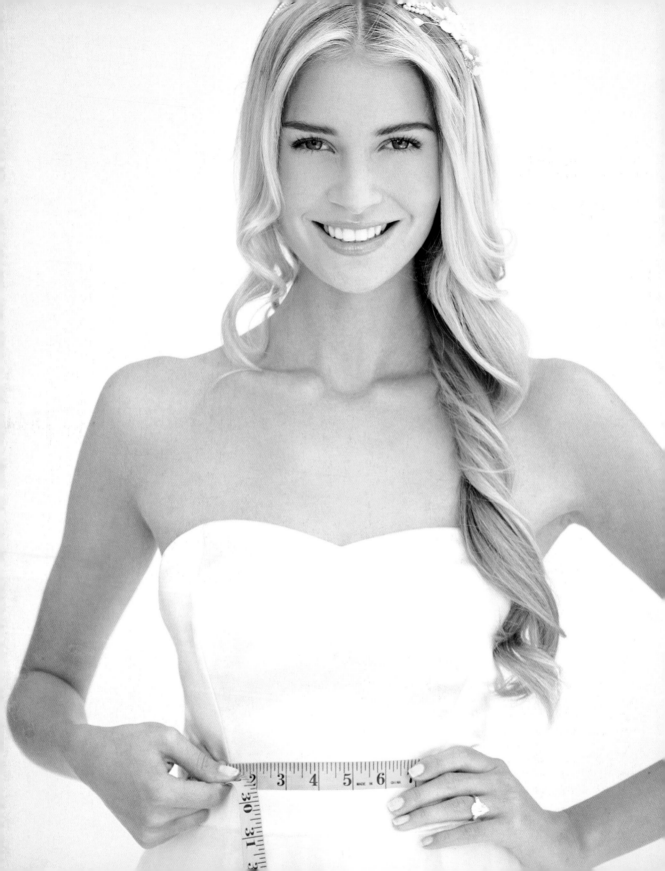

Slim & healthy

To get the best weight-loss and beauty benefits for your big day, combine your new exercise regime with a wholesome diet. In this chapter, we show you how to lose inches naturally while getting all the nutrients you need to feel well and full of energy. Discover how healthy your diet is with our self test, then use our fourteen-day diet plan to meet your target weight – without feeling deprived!

Why eat HEALTHILY?

*From helping you lose weight to boosting your energy,
a well-balanced diet is an essential part of your wedding preparations*

If you want to lose weight and look healthy, glowing and full of energy for your big day, ditch dieting for good and switch to a healthy eating regime. The simple fact is, faddy diets don't work. As well as being damaging to your health and looks – and seriously crippling to your bank balance – they fail to help you keep weight off in the long term because they only offer a quick-fix solution to weight-loss and don't teach you healthy eating habits. Once you've reached your target weight after weeks of deprivation, you start eating normally again and pile the pounds back on. It's no wonder recent research shows the average British woman starts three new diet regimes a year – if they worked, we'd only ever have to do one for life! If that's not enough to convince you to give good old-fashioned healthy eating a go, here are all the other reasons...

FUEL YOUR BODY
What you put into your body determines your entire wellbeing and affects how you feel and function. You might be tempted to restrict your diet and calorie intake, or you might have eaten poorly

for years, but either way, now is definitely the time to start nourishing your body properly – not restricting your dietary needs with low-calorie diets and juice cleanses that sap your energy. You need calories to keep your heart beating, mind alert and muscles working, and to give you the energy you need to get you through your wedding preparations and

{ *'The food you put into your body determines your entire wellbeing'* }

stick to your workouts – that means skipping meals is a definite no-no.

GET OPTIMUM HEALTH
Eating a healthy, balanced diet provides you with the nutrients needed to create new cells and regenerate your body, and helps maintain and strengthen bones, muscles and tendons. Good nutrition also regulates body processes such as

blood pressure, and can lower your risk of developing chronic diseases, including some cancers, heart disease, diabetes, high cholesterol and osteoporosis.

FEED YOUR LOOKS
The saying 'beauty comes from within' couldn't be more true. Eating a wide range of healthy foods full of vitamins, minerals and antioxidants nourishes your skin, hair and nails, so you glow from the inside out. Too much alcohol, caffeine, sugar, salt and other toxins burdens your organs, leaving you looking pasty and puffy, and triggering inflammation in the body – known to accelerate ageing.

MAINTAIN A HEALTHY WEIGHT
A healthy, balanced diet can help you lose weight at a sensible rate and then maintain it for life. Eating natural, wholesome foods including lean protein, fruit and vegetables, low-GI wholegrain varieties of carbohydrates and healthy fats – as opposed to convenience meals that are high in salt, sugar and unhealthy fats – will fill you up and ensure you get the nutrients you need. This way you'll lose weight slowly and steadily so you are more likely to keep the pounds off.

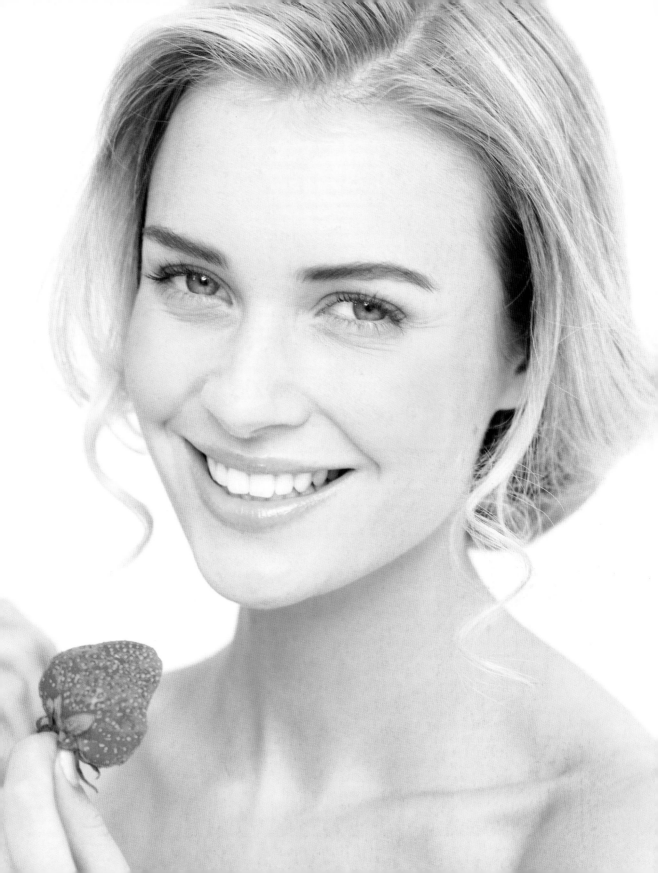

How good is YOUR DIET?

Take our nutrition test now to discover how healthy your diet is, and find out how you can improve your dietary intake

Think you're a healthy eater? You might need to think again. With our increasingly busy lifestyles, lack of home cooking and repeated use of processed foods, it has become all too easy for us to lose awareness of our diet. Take this test to see how healthy your diet actually is, and, if required, start making the changes you need to eat better, tastier and healthier food. Your wedding pics will show the difference!

Generally, how regularly do you eat a proper breakfast?
A Every day
B Most days
C Only at the weekend
D Hardly ever

How many servings of dairy (a glass of milk, a chunk of cheese or a pot of yoghurt counts as one; four cups of tea or coffee with milk or cereal with milk counts as half) do you eat each day?
A At least two servings
B One to two servings
C One serving
D Less than one

What proportion of the grain products you eat (breakfast cereals, pasta, bread, rice) are the high-fibre variety (wholegrain or wholemeal)?
A 100 per cent
B Half to three-quarters
C Less than half
D Hardly any

How many portions of fruit and vegetables do you eat per day?
A At least five
B Three to four
C One to two
D None to one

How often do you eat a portion of oily fish (fresh tuna, and fresh and canned salmon, sardines, mackerel, trout and herring)?
A At least twice a week
B About once a week
C Once or twice a month
D Rarely, or not at all

Which of the following best describes your biscuit/chocolate/cake/crisps eating habits?
A Less than once a week
B Once or twice a week
C Several times a week
D Almost every day

How often do you eat processed meats (for example, sausages, burgers, bacon, ham, pepperoni and paté)?
A Never, or less than once a week
B One to two times a week
C Three to five times a week
D Most days a week

How often do you eat takeaway or fast food?
A Less than once a month
B A couple of times a month
C One to two times a week
D Three or more times a week

How many cups of coffee do you drink daily?
A None to two
B Three to four

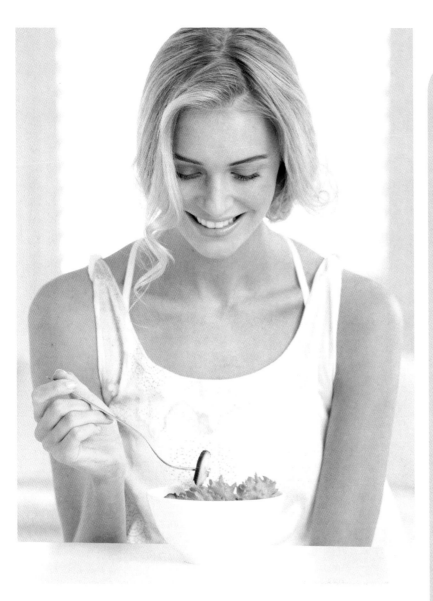

C Five to six
D More than six

How much water do you usually drink each day?
A At least 8 cups or glasses
B Six to seven cups or glasses
C Four to five cups or glasses
D Less than three cups or glasses

What best describes your alcohol-drinking habits (remember that one unit equals a small glass of wine, a half pint of beer or standard measure of spirits)?
A I drink one to two units regularly every day or don't drink at all
B I drink three to four units regularly every day
C I drink five to six units every day or have no more than three units most days but binge heavily (eight to 10 units) once a week
D I drink five to six units every day and usually binge heavily at least once a week as well

The results...

Mostly As...
HEALTHY, WELL-BALANCED DIET

Congratulations! You are eating a diet that's as balanced as most people find it practical to follow. Take care not to get too obsessed with eating healthily though, it's fine to relax from time to time and have a treat. There are no bad foods when they're eaten occasionally, only good and bad diets.

Mostly Bs...
HEALTHY, WELL-BALANCED DIET

You usually eat well within the recommended healthy eating guidelines, but there are some areas you could improve on. Watch your intake of fatty and sugary foods so your weight doesn't creep up. Filling up on vitamin-rich fruits and vegetables will make you less likely to give in to unhealthy treats.

Mostly Cs...
YOUR DIET COULD BE IMPROVED

Your diet isn't awful, but try to eat more fruit and veg, swap refined carbohydrates for wholegrains and replace fattier cuts of meat with leaner ones. Ditch processed foods and takeaways for tasty home-cooked versions, so you don't feel deprived.

Mostly Ds...
YOU ARE EATING A POOR DIET

You need to take action now to avoid storing up health problems for the future. Examine the reasons for your unhealthy habits: is a frantic lifestyle really a good enough reason not to eat well? Try our 14-day diet plan (page 62), to establish new eating habits.

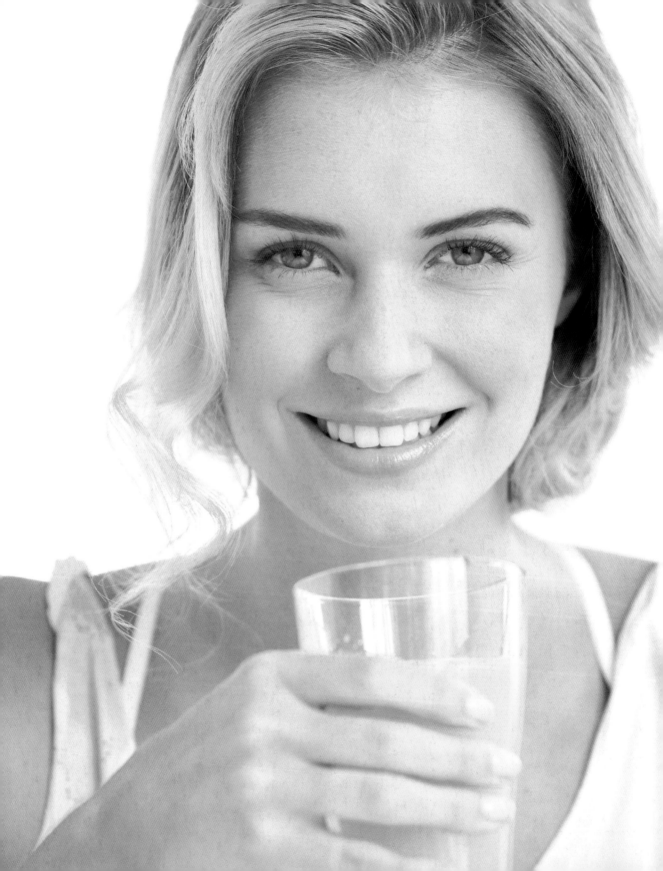

The healthy BASICS

*It's surprising the difference a few tweaks to your diet can make.
Give yourself a head start to looking good with these essential tips*

When you're trying to lose weight to look the best you can in your wedding dress, it can be easy to get obsessed with calorie-counting, measuring and weighing your food or thinking about what to eat and when. But the key to looking your best on your big day – and losing any excess pounds – is to start with a healthy, balanced diet. And that doesn't have to be complicated. Just follow our simple guidelines to keep you on track.

START RIGHT

Always eat breakfast. You've heard it a million times before, but eating breakfast is vital for keeping you slim. When you sleep, your blood-sugar levels drop as your body is effectively fasting. A good breakfast, combining protein and carbohydrates (for instance, porridge with nuts and seeds), will stop you snacking, and ensure you have the energy to get going. Remember the old adage of eating breakfast like a king,

lunch like a prince and supper like a pauper. Your stomach is most active first thing in the morning, when it functions more efficiently. As the 24-hour period goes on, it has less energy for digesting, and is more concerned with absorption and elimination, so keep meals light in the evening for maximum benefit.

> 'Studies show eating regularly is associated with a lower overall calorie intake'

EAT REGULARLY

Not eating enough can sabotage your weight-loss efforts just as much as overeating. When you reduce your food intake too much, your body holds on to the calories you consume and turns them to fat. Aim to eat three meals a day, along with a healthy, low-fat snack morning and afternoon. Studies show

that eating regularly is associated with a lower overall calorie intake, and your metabolic rate (the rate at which you burn calories) actually increases for a short period after eating a meal. Eating a meal or snack every three to four hours also helps keep your blood-sugar levels constant, so you avoid excess hunger or cravings that can make you want to fill up on the first high-fat, sugary foods you can get your hands on.

GO NATURAL

For optimum nutrition, choose natural, wholesome foods as often as possible. Swap refined carbohydrates, such as white bread, pasta and rice, for low-GI wholegrain varieties that contain more fibre to keep you fuller for longer, and eat plenty of protein, fruit and vegetables. Try to eat organic produce as often as possible for fewer additives to reduce the toxic load on your body and improve digestive function. Ditch processed foods and convenience meals which are often high in sugar, salt, unhealthy fats, chemicals and preservatives, as they can sabotage your weight-loss efforts. »

Fuel up!

~~~~~~~~~~~~~~~~~~~~~~~

Eat the right foods at the right times to boost your workouts and recover quickly.

To ensure you perform at your best and avoid fatigue when exercising, you need to start out with a 'full tank'. Eating (even if it's a healthy snack) every four hours is vital for active people. If you're exercising early in the morning, have a glass of juice or a banana before your workout, and don't skip breakfast afterwards. If you prefer to exercise later in the day, have a healthy snack about an hour before you work out, such as a banana, muesli bar, handful of dried fruit or a smoothie. And remember to drink plenty of water before and after your workout. Post-workout, you must rehydrate with water, then refuel by eating a healthy meal after. If your workout has lasted more than an hour, eat a healthy snack within half an hour of finishing to replenish your muscles' glycogen stores. Try a banana smoothie, a bowl of cereal or a couple of slices of wholemeal toast.

Instead, stock up on lots of healthy, portable snacks for taking with you on-the-go.

PROTEIN POWER

Aim to include protein at every meal. Vital for growth and repair, it helps you feel fuller for longer and, as your body has to work hard to digest protein, you'll boost your metabolic rate to burn more calories. Try to include some lean protein in every meal and snack. Good choices include lean meat, poultry or fish – a couple of portions of oily fish a week will ensure you get enough omega-3 – as well as beans, pulses, cheese, milk, tofu, nuts and seeds. And don't neglect eggs – they contain all eight essential amino acids and are a useful beauty food.

PORTION CONTROL

Eating the right foods is only half the story when it comes to weight-loss. Eating the right amount of food is just as important. A meat serving should be the size of a pack of cards, a pasta serving as big as your fist, and a serving of cheese the size of a matchbox. Try serving your food on a smaller plate (no bigger than 10 inches). Research shows you eat 25-35 per cent extra food when using a large plate. Aim to divide your plate in half and fill one side with non-starchy vegetables and salad, and the other into quarters, with one for carbohydrate-rich food (including starchy vegetables, such as potatoes) and the other for protein-rich foods.

STAY HYDRATED

Drink at least eight glasses of water a day. Not only is this essential to stay hydrated, it will help keep you feeling full, beat water retention and help your body metabolise stored fat. It's easy to confuse hunger with thirst and eat when what you really need is fluid. Make sure you drink extra water when you're exercising or in hot weather, to compensate for sweat loss and help you perform at your best. If you don't like water, add a slice of lemon or cucumber, or try naturally-hydrating coconut water.

'Include protein in every meal – it helps boost your metabolism'

SIX WAYS TO BEAT THE BLOAT

Learn which foods make you feel bloated, so you know what to avoid in the run-up to your wedding

HOLD THE SALT Water is attracted to sodium, so when you eat salty foods you retain fluid, leading to bloating and puffiness.

AVOID GASSY FOODS Some foods create more wind in your digestive tract than others, especially when eaten raw. These include beans and pulses, cauliflower, broccoli, Brussels sprouts, cabbage, onions, peppers and citrus fruits.

DON'T CHEW GUM While you chew, you swallow air, which gets trapped and causes bloating.

CUT DOWN ON FRIED FOODS Fatty foods, especially those that are fried, are digested more slowly, causing you to feel heavy and bloated.

SKIP SPICY FOODS Seasonings such as black pepper, chilli powder, hot sauces, onions, garlic and fresh chillies can speed up food transit time in the gut, which encourages wind.

DITCH THE FIZZY DRINKS Not only are they often laden with sugar, those bubbles can cause excess air in your digestive system.

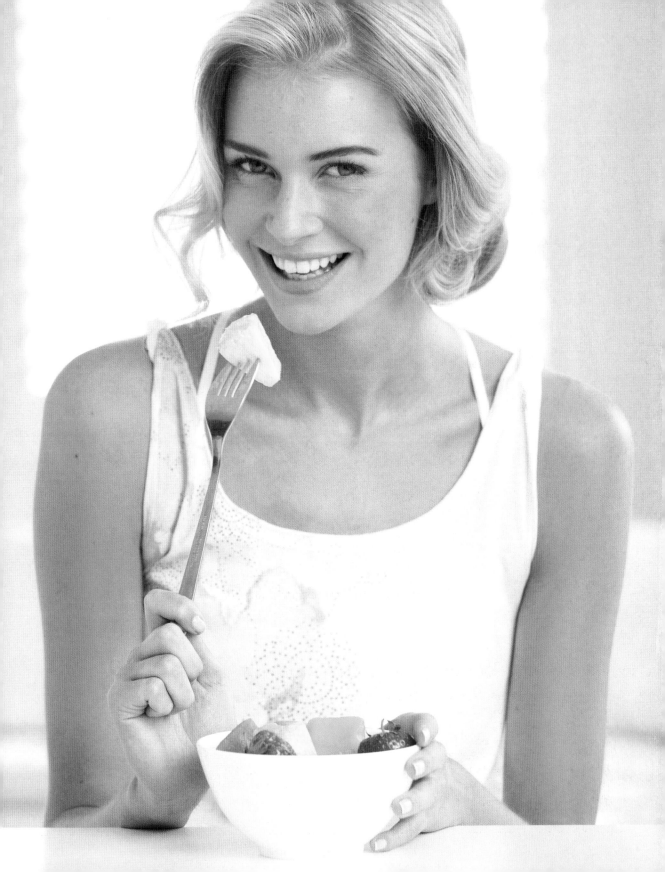

Weight-loss tips

As a bride-to-be, you have fantastic motivation to lose weight now, so make the most of the opportunity with our expert advice

The key to weight-loss success is to combine exercise with a healthy diet. There's no point in doing endless sit-ups or biceps curls if your muscles are hidden under a layer of flab!

The best way to lose weight is slowly and steadily. Studies show that a weight loss of 1-2lb (0.5-1kg) a week is the most effective way to lose weight and keep it off. You can do this by reducing the number of calories you eat or increasing the calories you burn. But the best way is to combine the two. Follow these easy steps to get slim and healthy.

1 WRITE IT DOWN
Keeping a food and mood diary is an important tool to help manage your relationship with food. Most of us don't think about what we are eating, or how all the things we unconsciously eat can add up – whether that's finishing off your child's leftovers, testing wedding cake or nibbling on canapés during engagement celebrations. Writing everything down (including snacks and drinks), and noting how you feel when you consume something, will help you become more aware of your eating patterns, and show you where you need to make changes to structure your lifestyle more effectively.

2 CHANGE YOUR EATING HABITS
Paying attention to what and how you eat will help you notice when you feel full and prevent overeating. Take time to chew every mouthful and taste what you are eating, rather than just guzzling it down! To help you learn to slow down, put down your cutlery after every mouthful and don't pick your knife and fork up until you've swallowed what's in your mouth. Also, avoid watching TV or reading while you eat.

> 'You eat 70 per cent more when you increase the variety of food on your plate'

3 KEEP IT SIMPLE
Make habit your friend. Diet plans sometimes have endless suggestions for meals and recipes that can get overwhelming. Instead, find what you like and stick with what works for you – at least until you get bored. Also, try to have a maximum of six types of food on your plate. Research shows you eat 70 per cent more when you increase

variety, as every new taste, texture and flavour re-stimulates your appetite. This is why breakfast cereals have so many ingredients now – to get you to eat more.

4 CUT OUT STIMULANTS
Speed up your weight-loss by reducing sugar in your diet. Not only is it linked to obesity, specifically belly fat, it also increases your risk of type 2 diabetes, hypertension and heart disease. And it's not just obvious sources you need to look out for, sugar is often found lurking in savoury sauces and low-fat foods. Try to avoid caffeine too – it has little nutritional value and can contribute to insulin resistance, making it harder for you to lose weight.

5 DON'T EMPTY YOUR PLATE
Try to always leave something on your plate, even if it's just a mouthful of food. This can help you break away from the idea that clearing your plate is a good thing – which is what we're often told when we're younger – and regain control over your eating. It'll give you the chance to sit back, listen to your body and decide if you're full or not. Eventually, you won't have to think so much about portion control because you'll only eat what your body needs. If you fight against leaving something on your plate,

you're probably one of the people who really needs to try doing it!

WEIGHTING GAME

6 If you have excess weight to shed, research now shows the best way to lose weight consistently is to reduce your calorie intake by 10 calories for every pound you want to lose permanently. So if you want to drop one stone, you'd need to cut your intake by 140 calories a day. You might have heard that cutting 500 calories a day was necessary for weight loss, but the new research reveals this will result in hitting a plateau before you reach your goal. While the downside of this news is that weight loss will take longer, on the positive side, you're more likely to stick to your new regime, and keep the weight off long term.

DON'T CRAVE IN

7 If cravings are your downfall, fret not. Try fighting your food urges the first time you get them – science shows the power of a craving dramatically decreases each time it comes back, so you may not even feel tempted the second or third time around. This approach might not work every time, but try to go from always giving in to giving in 20-30 per cent of the time.

SHOP SAVVY

8 Clear the junk food from your cupboards to avoid temptation at moments of low willpower, and restock them with healthy wholefoods. Avoid buying or eating from family-size bags of snacks (if you do, pour some into a bowl to prevent overeating) and, instead, buy single portions when shopping. It sounds obvious, but don't buy things you don't want to eat. If there's no chocolate in the house at

10pm, you're unlikely to go out to the corner shop to get some. When dining out, don't order supersize options, and if you can't resist a starter or dessert, share it with your partner or a friend.

COOK AT HOME

9 When you make your own food, you have control over the quality of ingredients and portion size. You'll also feel more connected to what you eat than if it was prepared by someone else. If you're short on time during the week, try cooking two meals at once so you spend less time in the kitchen, or prepare a big pot of wholegrains such as brown rice at the beginning of the week and use it in salads, toss with different spices or add toasted slivered nuts and dried fruits for super healthy and filling snacks. If you're too stressed or busy to think about making healthy packed lunches and dinners, then why not sign up for a home delivery service such as The Pure Package (purepackage.com) or Nosh Detox (noshdetoxdelivery.com), for yummy and nutritious meals that will help stop you falling off the wagon.

DRESS FOR SUCCESS

If you're trying to lose weight, buy a non-stretchy, form-fitting dress in the size you want to reach and hang it somewhere you'll see it every day. Regularly looking at it and remembering what it symbolises (your anticipated weight loss) will help focus your mind and keep your eye on the prize!

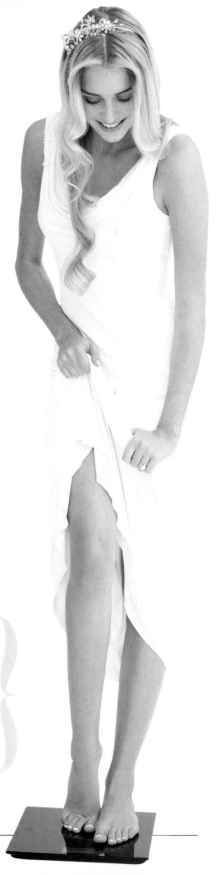

YOUR TWO-WEEK

Kick-start your healthy weight-loss plan, and see the pounds fall away

There are loads of diets to help you lose unwanted weight quickly. But if you want to drop the pounds and stay healthy, radiant and energised for good, you need a gentle approach. This 14-day plan is simple to follow, easy to fit into a busy lifestyle, and has all the nutrients you need for sustainable weight loss.

EAT FOR LIFE...

◆ **FEED YOUR BODY** with plenty of fruit (especially berries) and vegetables, oily fish, nuts, seeds and wholegrains.

◆ **AVOID REFINED CARBOHYDRATES** such as white flour, white pasta and sugar, as well as foods containing these.

◆ **AVOID BEIGE FOODS**, instead opting for colourful meals packed with goodness.

◆ **DRINK PLENTY OF WATER**, one or two cups of green tea daily and reduce alcohol.

◆ **AVOID PROCESSED FOODS**, aiming for at least 90 per cent of your diet to be home-made from fresh ingredients.

◆ **WHOLEGRAINS** such as oats, brown rice, pulses and beans keep you fuller for longer, so include plenty in your diet.

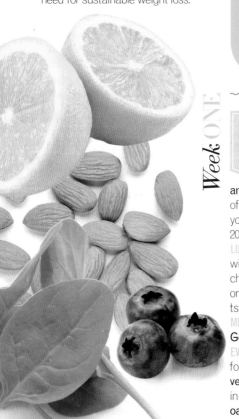

Week ONE

DAY 1

TO START Mug of **hot water** with a **slice of lemon**
BREAKFAST **Poached egg** on **rye toast.**
MID-MORNING SNACK **Blueberry and oat smoothie**, made with a handful of blueberries, 1 banana, 2-3 tbsp fat-free yoghurt, 1 tbsp oats, 1 tbsp flax oil and 200ml orange juice
LUNCH **Tuna and egg salad**, packed with green leaves, sugar-snap peas, cherry tomatoes, cucumber and red onion. Plus, 1 low-fat fruit **yoghurt** and 1 tsp **seed mix**
MID-AFTERNOON SNACK **The Food Doctor Get Set Bar** with a cup of **green tea**
EVENING MEAL Grilled **chicken** (make extra for tomorrow's lunch), steamed **green vegetables** and brown rice. Fresh fruit in season and 1 **Nairns** fruit or ginger oat biscuit

DAY 2

TO START **Lemon** drink
BREAKFAST **Porridge** made with skimmed or soya milk, a handful of **blueberries**, and a little **agave syrup**
MID-MORNING SNACK A handful of **almonds** and one or two pieces of **dark chocolate**
LUNCH **Wholemeal wrap**, filled with grilled **chicken**, grated **carrot**, baby leaf **spinach**, rocket and sun-dried **tomato**. Low-fat **fruit yoghurt** with 1 tsp **seed mix**
MID-AFTERNOON SNACK **Fruit** or **vegetable sticks**, and a cup of **green tea**
EVENING MEAL **Wholemeal spaghetti Bolognaise**, using **Quorn** or **turkey mince**. Follow your standard recipe but omit the wine. Add a carrot, 50g red lentils and some button mushrooms. **Stewed apple and blackberry** (with xylitol), topped with a handful of unsweetened **muesli**. Serve with fat-free Greek yoghurt

DAY 3

TO START **Lemon** drink
BREAKFAST Toasted **rye bread**, two grilled **tomatoes** and two slices of **lean ham**
MID-MORNING SNACK **Blueberry and oat smoothie**, as day 1
LUNCH **Carrot, lentil and tomato soup** (steam-fry ½ onion, add 1 chopped carrot, 50g puy lentils, ½ can chopped tomatoes and a handful chopped oregano. Simmer for 40 minutes) with **wholemeal pitta** stuffed with **humous** and **green salad leaves**. A handful of **almond** and **brazil nuts**, and one to two pieces of **dark chocolate**
MID-AFTERNOON SNACK Two **Nairns oatcakes** thinly spread with **peanut butter**, with a mug of **green tea**
EVENING MEAL Grilled **salmon** served with steamed **vegetables** and brown rice. **Fruit salad** with fat-free Greek yoghurt

DIET PLAN

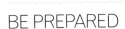

DAY 4

TO START **Lemon** drink
BREAKFAST As day 2
MID-MORNING SNACK Two **Nairns oat biscuits** with a mug of **green tea**
LUNCH One **wholemeal pitta** stuffed with slices of grilled **chicken**, grated **carrot**, spinach, rocket and cherry **tomatoes**. **Fat-free fruit yoghurt** mixed with 1 tsp seed mix
MID-AFTERNOON SNACK Two **Ryvita crackers** with **humous** and 1 **apple**
EVENING MEAL **Wholemeal pasta**, with tuna, cherry tomatoes, baby leaf spinach, handful of **basil leaves**, garlic and red onion. Fry the red onion and garlic in coconut oil. Drain the pasta and stir in all the ingredients. Heat for 3-5 minutes until combined before serving. One **meringue nest** filled with fat-free **yoghurt** and topped with fresh **fruit**

DAY 6

TO START **Lemon** drink
BREAKFAST As day 2
MID-MORNING SNACK Two **Nairns oat biscuits** with a cup of **green tea**
LUNCH Half a carton Covent Garden **Butternut squash and sweet potato soup** served with **wholemeal pitta** and **humous**. Handful of **almonds** and **brazil nuts** with one to two squares of **dark chocolate**
MID-AFTERNOON SNACK One **homemade cupcake**. Follow your usual recipe, but using wholemeal flour, xylitol and low-fat spread. Cup of **green tea**
EVENING MEAL Salmon fishcake, **superfood salad** (packed with leaves, fruit and veg) **brown rice** and **vegetable salad** (with onion, sweetcorn and peas). Make extra for tomorrow's lunch. One **sugar-free jelly** with fresh **fruit**

BE PREPARED

Spending a few hours planning your diet will make the changes so much easier. Here are some tips to help you.

PLAN YOUR SHOPPING Give yourself a helping hand by writing out a full shopping list before you go to the supermarket — and stick to it! Alternatively, order your groceries online as this keeps you focused and avoids impulse buys!

STOCK UP on healthy snacks such as oat and rice cakes, unsalted nuts, corn to make popcorn and a small amount of dark chocolate (at least 70 per cent cocoa solids). Fill your store-cupboard and fridge with humous (try different varieties, such as caramelised onion, pea and mint or sun-dried tomato) pulses, canned beans, brown rice, brown pasta, oats, skimmed milk, fat-free Greek yoghurt, fruit and veg, low-fat mature Cheddar, oily fish and eggs.

PLAN YOUR MEALS If you're too tired to cook after work, make your meals in advance — either in the slow cooker or even freeze some — much better than buying frozen ready meals!

CURB YOUR CRAVINGS Think about when you most want to eat 'bad' foods. A biscuit with your cuppa, a bar of chocolate mid afternoon when your energy is flagging, a little snack in front of the TV at night? Whenever it is, plan ahead. Have some healthy food swaps to hand and simply choose the wiser alternative.

THICK SOUPS are filling and nutritious, so make your own using homemade or low-salt stock. Add lean protein or pulses and beans to keep you fuller for longer. To preserve nutrients, cook, covered, on a low heat or use a slow cooker.

DAY 5

TO START **Lemon** drink
BREAKFAST One **boiled egg** with two slices of **wholegrain** toasted soldiers
MID-MORNING SNACK **Raspberry smoothie** made with handful of fresh or frozen **raspberries**, 2-3 tbsp fat-free **Greek yoghurt**, 200ml **orange juice**, one **banana**, 1 tbsp **flax oil**
LUNCH Carrot, lentil and tomato soup, as day 3, plus a **wholemeal pitta** spread with **humous**. Handful of **almonds** and a handful of berries
MID-AFTERNOON SNACK **The Food Doctor Get Set Bar** with a cup of **green tea**
EVENING MEAL Foil-wrapped **salmon fillet**, with **steamed green vegetables** and **new potatoes**. Place salmon on 2 slices of lemon, season, wrap and cook in a moderate oven for 15 minutes. **Stewed apple and blackberry**, as day 2

DAY 7

TO START **Lemon** drink
BREAKFAST ½ can of low-salt/low-sugar **baked beans** with 2 slices of **wholegrain** or **rye bread**
MID-MORNING SNACK **Blueberry & oat smoothie**, as day 1
LUNCH **Superfood** and **rice salads** with **tuna chunks**. One **cupcake**, as day 6
MID-AFTERNOON SNACK **The Food Doctor Get Set Bar** with a mug of **green tea**
EVENING MEAL **Chicken breast**, stuffed with **low-fat cheese spread** and fresh chopped **chilli** and fresh **herbs** of your choice, baked for 20 minutes in a moderate oven. Served with **green vegetables** and **mashed carrots** and **sweet potato**. **Baked apple** stuffed with **berries**, sweetened with xylitol or agave syrup, served with a dollop of **fat-free yoghurt**

YOUR TWO-WEEK DIET PLAN *CONT...*

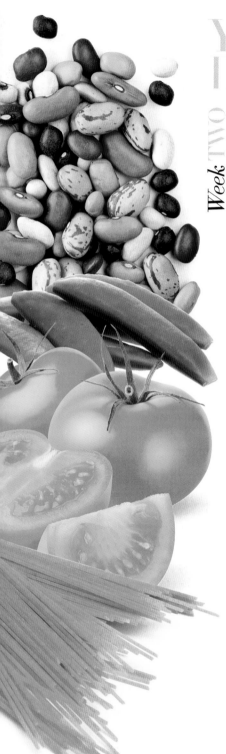

Week TWO

DAY 8

TO START Lemon drink
BREAKFAST Toasted rye bread, 2 grilled tomatoes and 2 slices of lean ham
MID-MORNING SNACK Handful of almonds, one to two pieces of dark chocolate and a cup of green tea
LUNCH Healthy BLT. Grilled very lean bacon, green salad leaves (rocket, spinach leaves and lettuce), sliced tomatoes and a dash of lowest-fat mayonnaise in wholegrain bread or rye. One pot of fat-free yoghurt mixed with 1 tsp seed mix
MID-AFTERNOON SNACK Two wholemeal or Ryvita crackers with humous. One apple
EVENING MEAL One salmon fish cake, served with superfood salad and sweet potato wedges. Stewed apple and blackberry, as day 2

DAY 9

TO START Lemon drink
BREAKFAST Porridge, as day 2
MID-MORNING SNACK The Food Doctor Get Set Bar
LUNCH Carrot, lentil and tomato soup as day 3, with wholemeal pitta stuffed with humous. One low-fat fruit yoghurt mixed with 1 tsp seed mix and one to two pieces of dark chocolate
MID-AFTERNOON SNACK Two Nairns oat biscuits with a mug of green tea
EVENING MEAL Chilli con carne made to your standard recipe, with very lean beef or turkey mince or Quorn, chopped peppers, celery and mixed beans. Serve with brown rice. One meringue nest filled with fruit and low-fat yoghurt

DAY 10

TO START Lemon drink
BREAKFAST Boiled egg with 2 slices of toasted wholegrain or rye soldiers
MID-MORNING SNACK Handful of almonds and brazil nuts. One cup of green tea
LUNCH Wholemeal wrap, as day 2 Low-fat fruit yoghurt mixed with 1 tsp seed mix
MID-AFTERNOON SNACK Two wholemeal bread sticks, vegetable sticks and humous dip
EVENING MEAL Wholemeal spaghetti, with green pesto, chopped asparagus, soya beans, red onion, pine nuts and spinach leaves, served with 25g crumbled, low-fat feta. One pot sugar-free jelly served with fresh fruit and one to two pieces of dark chocolate

DAY 11

TO START Lemon drink
BREAKFAST Toasted rye bread, 2 grilled tomatoes and 2 slices of lean ham
MID-MORNING SNACK Blueberry & oat smoothie, as day 1
LUNCH Vegetable and bean soup (steam-fy ½ onion. Add 1 sliced parsnip, 1 chopped potato, 100g French beans, small can butter beans and 300g vegetable stock, simmer for 20 minutes and sprinkle with parsley). Serve with wholemeal pitta and humous.
MID-AFTERNOON SNACK Two Nairns oat biscuits with a mug of green tea
EVENING MEAL Baked salmon on a bed of brown rice and vegetables stir-fried in coconut oil. Stewed rhubarb (sweetened with xylitol), topped with unsweetened muesli and served with a dollop of fat-free Greek yoghurt

DAY 12

TO START **Lemon** drink
BREAKFAST **Porridge**, as day 2
MID-MORNING SNACK Handful of **almonds** and **brazil nuts**, with 2 pieces of **dark chocolate**
LUNCH **Tuna salad**, 2 **Ryvita crackers** with **humous**. One low-fat **fruit yoghurt** mixed with 1 tsp of **seed mix**
MID-AFTERNOON SNACK **The Food Doctor Get Set Bar** with a mug of **green tea**
EVENING MEAL **Vegetable and chickpea casserole**. Steam-fry ½ onion and 1 clove garlic. Add ½ courgette, ½ red pepper, ½ butternut squash and sauté for five minutes. Add ½ can chopped tomatoes and ½ can chickpeas, and simmer for 30 minutes. Top with flat-leaf parsley and serve with **brown rice**. One **baked apple** filled with chopped dates, and **fat-free Greek yoghurt**

'Help me, I'm hungry!'

There are plenty of foods you can eat that won't pile on the pounds

◆ **FRUIT AND VEGETABLES** are unlimited (white potatoes are starch, so don't fill up too much on these – swap for antioxidant-rich sweet potatoes).
◆ **POPCORN** is easy to make. Just place the corn in a saucepan, close the lid, turn up the heat and wait for them to start popping! Sprinkle with some xylitol if you like them sweet.
◆ **BROWN RICE** is packed with nutrients and fills you up too – you can eat as much as you like.
◆ **PULSES AND BEANS** keep you fuller for longer and maintain your energy levels (as well as being a great source of

nutrients and fibre). Pop them into homemade soups, add to casseroles, or add to canned tomatoes, onions and herbs for a hearty (wholemeal) pasta sauce.
◆ **FANCY SOMETHING SWEET?** If you are a bit of a baker, make cakes or cupcakes, but replace the sugar with xylitol, use wholemeal self-raising flour and a low-fat margarine.
◆ **AVOID BUTTER ICING.** Warm cakes, especially spicy versions, are lovely with a dollop of 0 per cent fat Greek yoghurt. Grate an apple and add some seed mix. This is very nutritious and fills you up, and gives you a sweet hit when you need it.

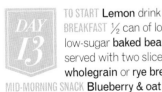

DAY 13

TO START **Lemon** drink
BREAKFAST ½ can of low-salt, low-sugar **baked beans** served with two slices of **wholegrain** or rye bread
MID-MORNING SNACK **Blueberry & oat smoothie**, as day 1
LUNCH **Wholemeal wrap**, as day 2. **Low-fat fruit yoghurt** mixed with 1 tsp **seed mix**
MID-AFTERNOON SNACK Two **Nairns oat biscuits** with a mug of **green tea**
EVENING MEAL **Grilled salmon** served with steamed vegetables and **brown rice**. Fresh fruit salad with a dollop of **fat-free Greek yoghurt**

DAY 14

TO START **Lemon** drink
BREAKFAST **Porridge** as day 2
MID-MORNING SNACK Two **Nairns oat biscuits** with a mug of **green tea**
LUNCH **Healthy BLT**, as day 8 One pot of **fat-free yoghurt** mixed with 1 tsp **seed mix**
MID-AFTERNOON SNACK Two **wholemeal** or **Ryvita crackers** with **humous**. One **apple**
EVENING MEAL **Spaghetti Bolognaise**, served with wholemeal spaghetti, as day 2. One pot of low-fat, low-sugar **chocolate mousse**

SLIMMING GOOD SWAPS

SUGAR Replace with xylitol or stevia to keep blood sugar balanced. Both are lower in calories and can be used in baking for sin-free cakes!
OIL Fill a spray can with olive oil and use when cooking. For an even healthier choice, swap for coconut oil. Use flax oil in salad dressing.
CREAM Fat-free Greek yoghurt will become your best friend. Use it in cooking, add some vanilla extract to make a lovely sweet and creamy alternative to cream.
MEAT Avoid too much red meat – it's laden with unhealthy saturated fats. If you like mince, opt for chicken, or even better, turkey mince. Quorn mince is also a great substitute, and a whooping 70 per cent less saturated fat.
BISCUITS Love a biscuit with your cuppa? For a low-GI treat, try Nairns Oat Biscuits with ginger, fruit and spice or mixed fruit.

This diet plan is created by Sarah Flower, a nutritionist and author of several recipe books, including *The Healthy Lifestyle Diet Cookbook*, (How To Books, £14.99). Sarah is passionate about healthy eating for all the family. She likes to adapt family favourites and give them a healthy twist, creating healthy cakes and desserts. For more information, visit sarahflower.co.uk.

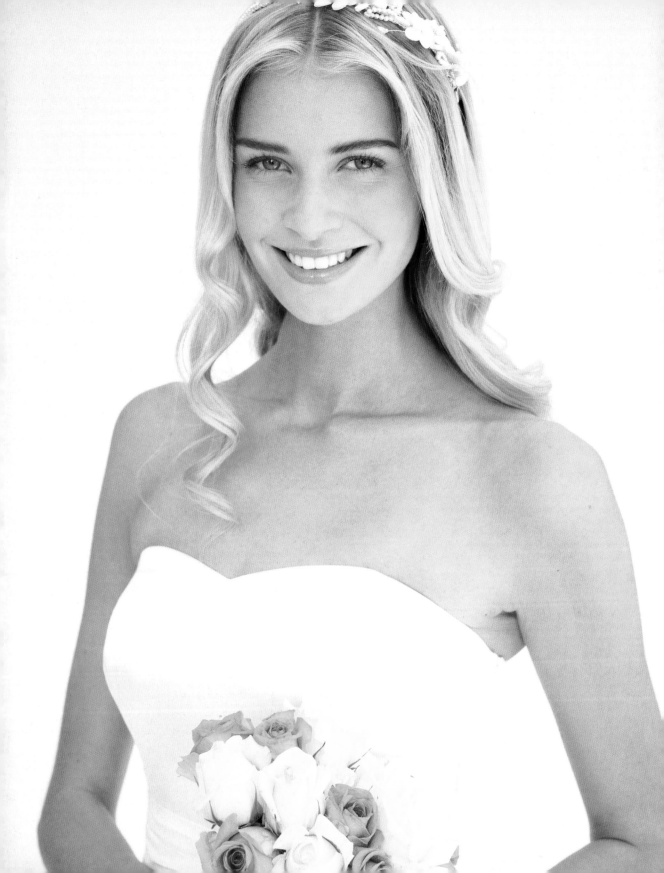

Beautiful you

It's time to get glowing and gorgeous for your big day! For radiant skin, lustrous hair, a dazzling smile and a fabulous body from top to toe, read on to discover our hassle-free grooming tips and perfect pampering ideas. Plus, we'll show you the beauty superfoods that'll help you feel gorgeous from the inside out, and provide planning advice to take the stress out of looking 100 per cent picture perfect - whatever stage you're at in your wedding preparations.

Get radiant skin

You're going to be a beautiful, blushing bride — not a spotty one. Follow these skincare rules for a smooth, flawless complexion on your wedding day

There's nothing more flattering than the glow of natural happiness that a bride exudes. To help that glow along, the secret is all in the planning. Leave your grooming too late and you could be setting yourself up for all kinds of disasters – such as breakouts and allergic reactions – when you're trying to look serene and poised. But fear not: whether you have six months or six weeks to go, we've got the advice you need to get gorgeous skin.

PERFECT YOUR SKINCARE

Get going with our regime, for skin that's healthy and glowing.

Just as your body needs a regular fitness programme to stay trim and toned, your complexion requires a dedicated approach, with a cleansing and moisturising regime to rid your skin of impurities and keep it hydrated.

Good products help, but it's more important that the ones you use are suitable for your skin type (oily, combination, normal or sensitive) and age-appropriate, so your skin gets exactly what it needs. If you're thinking about changing the brand, or types of products you use, do it at least a month before your wedding, as introducing new products can lead to allergic reactions, dryness, oiliness and other side effects that take time to correct. Many skincare counters offer skin analysis to help pinpoint the right products for your needs, but do try to keep things as simple as possible – less really is more when it comes to products, and there's no point using 10 when three will do. This will help prevent your skin from looking and feeling 'overloaded'. Once you've settled on your products, you need to use them regularly, morning and night (and yes, that means no sleeping in your make-up) to get maximum benefits.

CLEANSING

A good cleanse is essential to remove make-up residue, dirt and grime and to shift dead cells and sebum. Apply your cleanser to dry skin, using a light circular massage to bring fresh blood to the surface and reduce puffiness. Products with a lathering quality tend to be harsh on your skin. Try nourishing cream cleansers instead, to keep your skin hydrated. Soaps are definitely out.

TONING

A gentle sweep of toner across your face will help remove those last few traces of cleanser, and refresh and hydrate your skin. Avoid alcohol-based products – it's better to go for natural, nutrient-rich ingredients, such as aloe vera, cucumber, calendula and rosewater.

MOISTURISING

Your skin contains a natural lipid barrier to protect it against the elements and dirt. By applying a moisturiser, you enhance the strength of your skin's shield, and preserve the hydration levels in its deep layers. Choose a protective SPF day cream and an intensive moisturiser or face oil at night. Even if you think your skin is oily, moisturising is essential – use lighter products based on plant oils, so your complexion doesn't get congested. A moisturiser or foundation with a broad-spectrum SPF15 protection will help prevent UV damage and slow skin ageing. Added antioxidants are a bonus too. And remember to apply it to your lips and neck. Use a stronger sunscreen if you're outside a lot.

EXFOLIATION

Gentle exfoliation will speed up your skin's cellular turnover, but steer clear of abrasive, grainy products as they can damage sensitive skin. Using a soft muslin cloth is ideal, or, for a thorough occasional exfoliation, choose products that contain alpha hydroxy acids (AHAs), chemical compounds found in citric fruits and cane sugar that act as a natural exfoliant. Or pick products containing fine jojoba beads. How often you should use them depends on your skin type, but start with once or twice a week. If your skin still appears dull or flaky, use more regularly. »

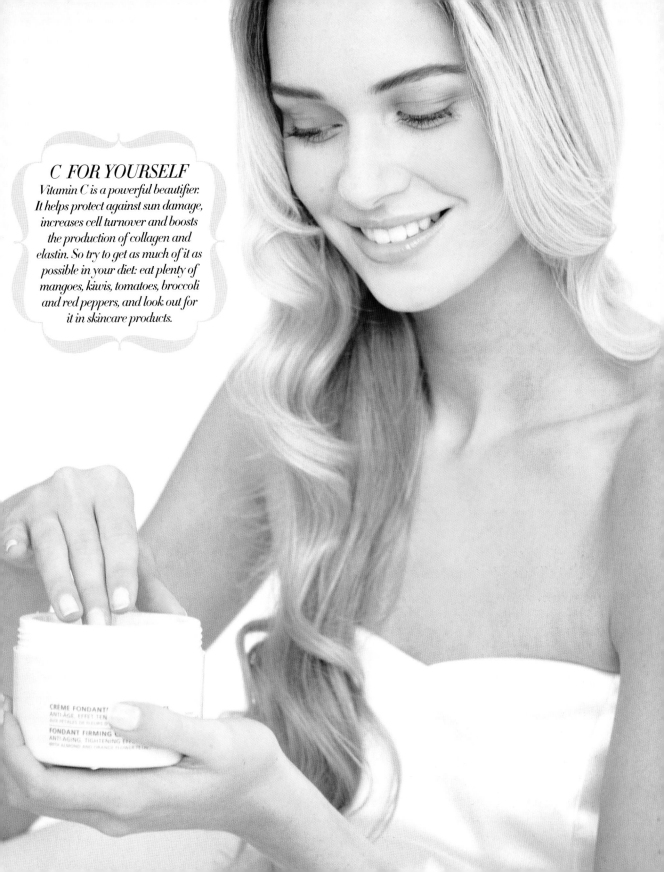

C FOR YOURSELF

*Vitamin C is a powerful beautifier.
It helps protect against sun damage,
increases cell turnover and boosts
the production of collagen and
elastin. So try to get as much of it as
possible in your diet: eat plenty of
mangoes, kiwis, tomatoes, broccoli
and red peppers, and look out for
it in skincare products.*

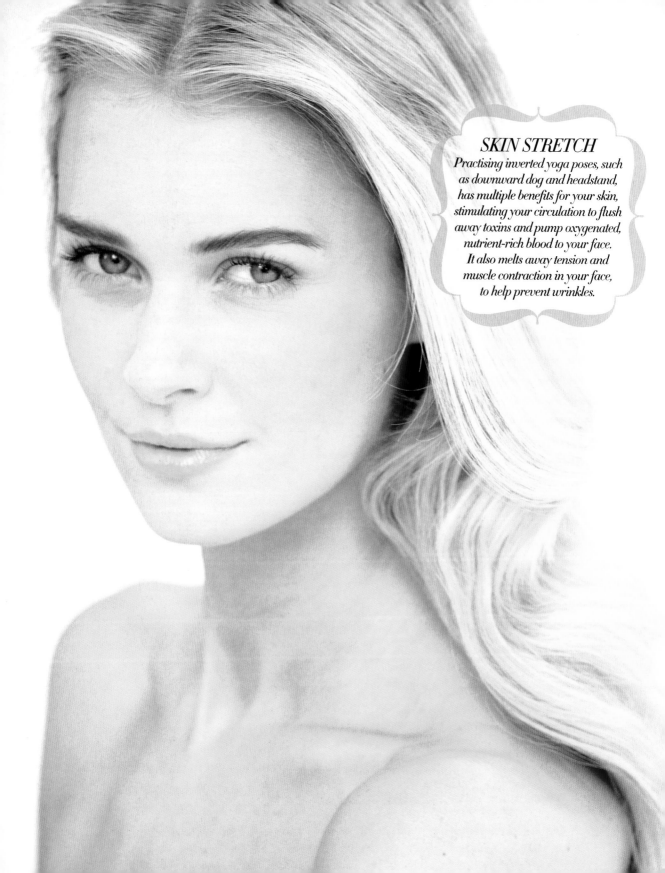

SKIN STRETCH

Practising inverted yoga poses, such as downward dog and headstand, has multiple benefits for your skin, stimulating your circulation to flush away toxins and pump oxygenated, nutrient-rich blood to your face. It also melts away tension and muscle contraction in your face, to help prevent wrinkles.

LOOK AT YOUR LIFESTYLE

Having great skin isn't just about slathering the latest cream onto your face. What you put into your body and how you live your life are equally crucial.

GET LOTS OF SLEEP

A regular eight hours is essential for a glowing complexion: your body produces more protein when you sleep, allowing the skin's cells to renew and repair the damage caused by ultraviolet rays, pollution and toxins. It also increases human growth hormone production, to retain skin elasticity for fewer wrinkles. You'll also help prevent bloodshot eyes, bags and dark under-eye circles.

DRINK WATER

Drinking the recommended eight glasses of water every day will help your skin to rehydrate and flush out any toxins in the body for clearer, fresher and plumper skin. If you're exercising, you need to up your water intake to replace fluids lost when you sweat. Hydrate before you start to exercise; sip water during the session and then rehydrate afterwards. In daily life, try switching from tea and coffee to herbal blends and juices.

EXERCISE MORE

As well as giving your circulation a massive boost for a healthy glow, exercise also encourages your body to flush away toxins. Half an hour's gentle exercise a day can make a massive improvement.

SMOKING

A nicotine habit can add years to your appearance. Smoking deprives your skin of oxygen, leaving it looking dull and dowdy, and reduces the skin's collagen levels (due to the toxins cigarette smoke contains), causing your skin to age. Ask your GP for advice on quitting.

ALCOHOL

Too much boozing affects your looks in the short and long term. The morning after, you can expect to look bloated, puffy, pale and tired, because booze affects your quality of sleep, weakens your immune systems and deprives the skin of hydration, vitamins and nutrients. It also dilates the small blood vessels in the skin, which can lead to permanent redness. To achieve a radiant complexion, you should reduce your alcohol intake – and try to avoid it entirely in the week running up to your wedding.

Nature knows best

Products with natural ingredients will keep your skin peachy and pure

Natural skincare has come a long way, and products from brands such as Elemis, Neal's Yard and Dr Hauschka – which combine scientific innovations with pure, plant-based ingredients – are often as effective as their synthetic counterparts. These products are free from chemicals such as parabens and sulphates, which can irritate the skin, and their natural ingredients also combat ageing. These include antioxidant vitamins A, C and E, which fight the free radicals involved in inflammation and ageing inside the body, and help battle acne and wrinkles on the outside. They also include superfood berries such as goji and açai (and the more familiar rosehip and blueberry), which are rich in antioxidant vitamins; soothing herbs, such as chamomile and calendula for inflamed skin; and natural plant oils, such as jojoba and argan, which are similar to the skin's oil, and so more easily absorbed into its deeper layers. They also contain essential oils such as lavender and frankincense, which provide heavenly scents without the chemical load.

EAT YOURSELF BEAUTIFUL

Enhance your looks the natural way with these beautifying superfoods

PRAWNS, SALMON AND LOBSTER Their pinkness is due to the antioxidant astaxanthin, which is shown to improve skin elasticity.

MACKEREL AND TUNA They're rich in omega-3 fatty acids, which keep your skin supple, and selenium, which fights ageing free radicals.

BLUEBERRIES Their antioxidant properties protect against premature ageing.

SPINACH It contains lutein, which keeps your eyes healthy and sparkling.

WALNUTS AND ALMONDS They're packed with protein, and rich in omega-3 fatty acids, to give you smoother skin, healthier hair and brighter eyes.

KIWIS, LEMONS AND ORANGES They're loaded with vitamin C and antioxidants to prevent wrinkles, protect against sun damage and reduce scars.

TOMATOES AND RED PEPPERS They contain the antioxidant lycopene, which is shown to protect against sun damage.

TOFU AND EDAMAME They're rich in isoflavones, which improve skin elasticity and reduce wrinkles.

EGGS A great source of protein and omega-3 fatty acids, which prevent skin-ageing; they also contain the amino acid cystine, which helps form collagen.

Healthy HAIR

Your hair will be your crowning glory on the big day. But first you'll need to plan your style, nurture your locks and refine your look. Here's how you do it

Nobody wants a bad hair day, especially when it's their wedding! Your hair is a reflection of your inner health, which comes from your diet and lifestyle, and also your personality. For shiny and stylish locks that suit you perfectly and make you feel amazing on your big day, use these fabulous haircare and grooming tips.

ARRIVE IN STYLE

You need to work with your hairdresser well in advance to find the right style for your type of hair and face-shape. If you are considering a drastic restyle, make sure you try it months before the wedding, so there's time to remedy mistakes. Once you've settled on a style, you should work with your stylist to refine it, so it complements your dress and make-up. Trim your hair every six weeks, to keep split-ends at bay and your hair in tip-top condition, and have a final trim a week before your wedding.

FIND YOUR SHADE

Your hair colour is just as important as your hairstyle, and if you're thinking of going for a dramatic change, you may need a few appointments to perfect your shade. Ask your hairdresser to recommend colours that will work with your skin tone (generally around two or three shades lighter or darker than your natural hair colour) and highlight your eye colour. Keep newly coloured hair glossy and rich with Philip Kingsley's Pre-Shampoo Elasticizer, which is formulated to deliver moisture inside the hair's cuticle, boosting suppleness, bounce and strength without fading your colour. If you're heading off for a honeymoon in the sun, don't have your hair coloured the week before the ceremony; instead ask your stylist for a clear-gloss treatment that'll leave your hair super-shiny in bright sunshine.

> *'Your perfect style will suit your face and hair type — and reflect your personality'*

KEEP IT CONDITIONED

Colouring, styling, sun exposure and heat damage can all take their toll on your hair, so keep it in top condition with a nourishing hair treatment once a month. Comb a mask through your hair, wrap it up in a towel and leave it to work for 10 to 15 minutes. For general cleansing, experts say you should wash your hair whenever you feel you need to, massaging your scalp as you shampoo to stimulate blood flow and encourage the growth of healthy hair. If your hair is exposed to the elements, shield it with a UV protector such as Schwarzkopf Bonacure Sun Protect UV Protection Spray, and use a heat protection spray, such as Kérastase Nutritive Nectar Thermique before blow-drying and straightening. And avoid conditioning your hair on the big day – your stylist will need total control of your hair and can add shine and condition with their other products.

FIND THE PERFECT STYLE

The best bridal style is one that suits your face and hair type, and reflects your personality. So stay true to you and don't be bullied into stereotypical wedding styles like up-do's and ringlets if they make you feel uncomfortable – on your wedding day, above all others, you'll want your hair to make you feel confident. Find a hairdresser who specialises in dressing bridal hair (ask to see their portfolio) and meet them in advance, so there's plenty of time for trial and error. Take along pictures of styles you like and any tiaras or veils you intend to wear, and take photos to ensure your style works from all angles. And have a dry-run before the big day, to see how long it'll take to get your hair looking lustrous and lovely. Because you don't want to be late to the altar…

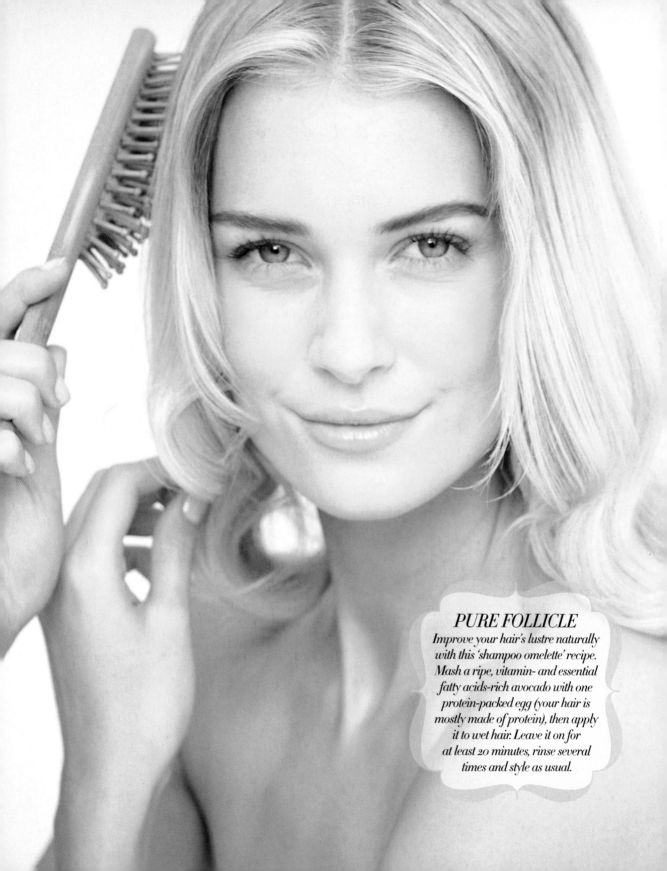

PURE FOLLICLE

Improve your hair's lustre naturally with this 'shampoo omelette' recipe. Mash a ripe, vitamin- and essential fatty acids-rich avocado with one protein-packed egg (your hair is mostly made of protein), then apply it to wet hair. Leave it on for at least 20 minutes, rinse several times and style as usual.

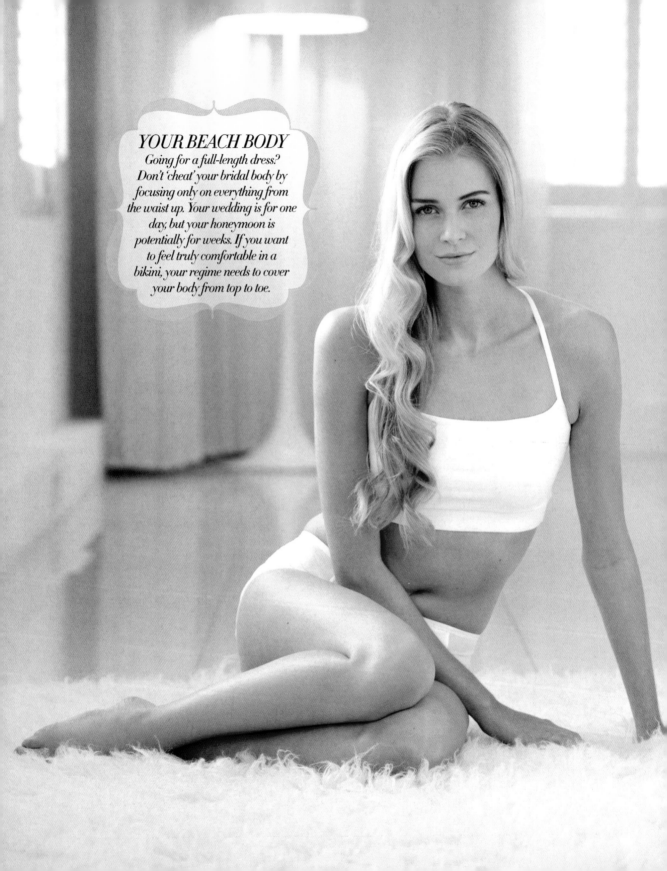

YOUR BEACH BODY

Going for a full-length dress?
Don't 'cheat' your bridal body by
focusing only on everything from
the waist up. Your wedding is for one
day, but your honeymoon is
potentially for weeks. If you want
to feel truly comfortable in a
bikini, your regime needs to cover
your body from top to toe.

Bridal BODY

These are the salon treatments and home-pampering methods you need for a beautifully toned, tanned and buffed-to-perfection body

You're most likely going to arrive at your wedding sheathed in shimmering silk and with your hair primped and teased to perfection – and the last thing you want is to let your look down with dull, dowdy skin. A glowing, toned body can easily be yours – just follow these rules and use these expert tips to achieve salon-quality skin tone.

USE A BODY BRUSH

Daily body brushing is an inexpensive and easy way to stimulate your circulation and lymphatic system. It'll help eliminate toxins, reduce the appearance of cellulite and remove dead skin cells, to get your skin glowing and revitalised.

Look for a brush with firm, natural bristles and a long handle, so you can get to hard-to-reach places. Before you shower, sweep the brush over every surface of your body (avoiding delicate areas) using long, firm strokes. Begin at your feet and work your way upwards, always brushing towards the heart.

Start off with gentle strokes, then do it a bit harder after a few weeks to get more benefits. If you need extra exfoliation on problem areas such as the knees, elbows and feet, use exfoliating mitts in the shower with a moisturising

shower wash for smooth, supple skin, or a specific body exfoliating product, such as Clinique Sparkle Skin Body Exfoliator.

MOISTURISE EVERY DAY

While drinking plenty of water hydrates your skin from within, regular moisturising will keep it soft, smooth and supple on the outside.

From lotions and oils to butters and balms, the range of moisturisers can be overwhelming, so we recommend that you choose one that has an aroma you

> { *'Regular moisturising will keep your skin soft, smooth and supple'* }

really like, so you're more likely to slather it on and reap the benefits.

Avoid putting more toxins into your body by using organic moisturisers from Organic Surge or Green People, and look for products that use lots of natural ingredients such as plant oils. We like Spatopia's Argan Body Butter – argan oil is a rich source of vitamin E and omega-3 essential fatty acids that

reduces wrinkles and inflammation, and improves elasticity. We also like Origins Ginger Souffle Whipped Body Cream, with nourishing olive oil, grape seed oil and apricot kernel oil.

CHOOSE FAKE TAN

There's nothing like a gorgeous, glowing tan to set off that stunning white dress. And while a tan from sun exposure is often the most natural-looking, we all know that the damage UV rays cause to our skin just isn't worth it – which is why fake tan is the safest way to go.

But it's not always the easiest thing to get right. A fake tan disaster is bad news at any time, but on one of the most important days of your life? You don't want to look at your wedding photos for years to come and cringe at your orange glow, blotchy hands or streaky arms.

Preparation is key to successful tanning. If you're exfoliating and moisturising as above (paying special attention to dry areas, such as your ankles, elbows and wrists where tanner can collect), that's half the battle won, as your skin will be perfectly primed. You also need to decide whether you'll be self-tanning or having salon treatments. If it's the former, you should experiment with different products (try BeauBronz, Famous Dave, FakeBake and St. Tropez) to find the shade that suits you, and ➤➤

then practise, practise, practise. Try out the various application methods (hands, tanning mitts or latex gloves) and learn how to spread the tan evenly. If you don't feel confident with self-tanning, it's worth splashing out on a professional salon tan (try St.Tropez, Elemis, Decléor or Fantasy Tan). Just make sure you have a trial run so you know you're happy with the shade, scent and application.

For your big day, tan a few days beforehand so you have time to sort out any disasters, allow the colour to develop properly and prevent it from rubbing off on your dress.

PAMPER HANDS AND FEET

Your hands need to look their best when you're flashing your wedding ring to everyone, and you'll want your feet to look pretty on your honeymoon. Having regular manicures and pedicures every few weeks in the run-up to your ceremony will ensure your skin and nails look flawless, and you should have your final mani/pedi the day before the wedding – just allow a good few hours to let the polish dry and stay smudge-free. If you're considering nail extensions, have

a trial run so you can get used to them. At home, moisturise your hands daily and rub in cuticle oil regularly; and soak feet twice a week in warm water and a few drops of revitalising peppermint to keep them feeling fresh. Try a little extra TLC with a deep-conditioning treatment such as Bliss's Glamour Gloves and Softening Socks – they have self-activating hydrating gel linings impregnated with natural moisturisers.

GET SILKY SMOOTH SKIN

If you're self-conscious about body or facial hair, you need to take action. Shaving and bleaching might suffice normally but if you don't want to be worrying about hairs showing up in your photos, or grooming on your honeymoon, you should invest in more effective methods. If you've ever considered permanent hair removal, now's the time to splash out, but remember that intense pulsed light and laser treatments require up to six sessions over an eight-month period to really work. Waxing is a cheaper but good alternative way of staying hair-free. If you're a 'waxing virgin' or have had a long break from

waxing, start having regular treatments three months before your big day. And make your final defuzzing appointment three days before the wedding, so your skin has time to recover.

FIRM YOUR BODY

If your wobbly bits need extra help, why not treat yourself to a non-invasive body-toning treatment? There are tons of highly effective treatments to try, for

> *'There are plenty of effective treatments if your wobbly bits need toning up'*

instance body wraps such as Universal Contour Wrap, which guarantees a loss of at least six inches from all over the body in one session (universalcontourwrap.com).

Ultrasound treatments also work well: MedContour aids lymphatic drainage and is perfect for targeting problem areas such as saddlebags and muffin tops (med-contour.co.uk).

Radio frequency treatments can also work well: Thermage tightens, contours and smooths the body as well as stimulating your body's renewal of collagen (thermage.com).

And if all this seems a bit science-fiction, good old-fashioned massage can do wonders for your skin tone and firmness. We recommend Elemis' Body Sculpting & Colon Therapy massage to reduce bloating and firm the body, and Bliss Spa's Arm Candy treatment to banish bingo wings.

HERE COMES THE SUN BLOCK

Strap marks? No way! SPF cream will banish them from your wedding photos

Now you have your fake tanning regime in place, there's absolutely no reason you should expose your body to harmful UV rays without effective sun protection. In the run-up to your wedding, the last thing you'll want is dodgy tan lines on your arms, chest and back that could end up showing up in your photos. To make sure you prevent it, follow a sensible daily routine and take the time to apply a high-SPF cream to any areas that will be exposed to the sun at the start of the day –

especially face, neck, shoulder and hands – and top up at regular interval through the day.

The same applies if you're heading off for a pre-wedding sunshine getaway with your hens – even if you dare to go topless for an alluring all-over tan, you still need to protect your skin. This will not only to avert sunburn, which could bring your hen night antics down to earth with a bump, but also prevent irreversible skin damage and premature ageing.

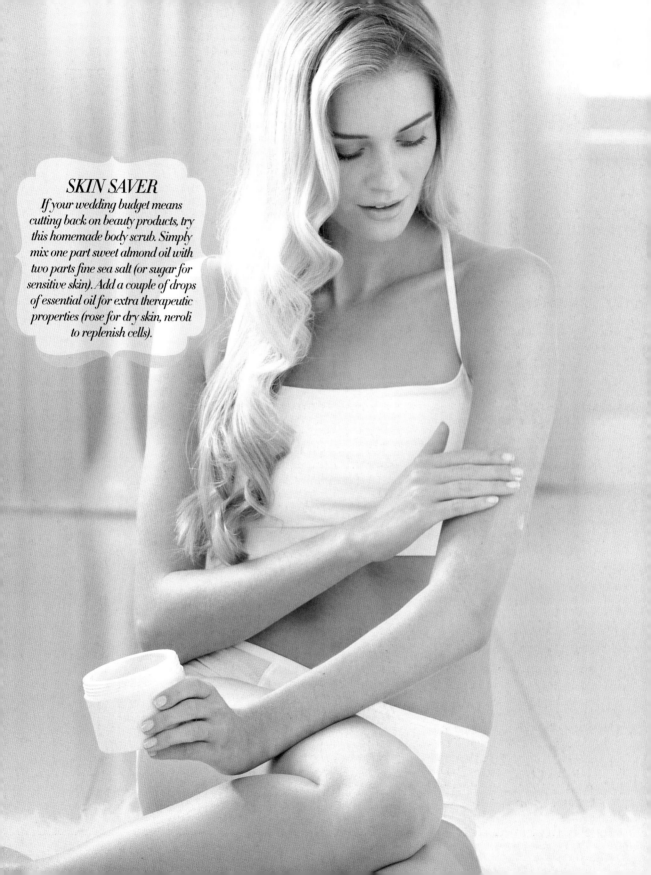

SKIN SAVER

If your wedding budget means cutting back on beauty products, try this homemade body scrub. Simply mix one part sweet almond oil with two parts fine sea salt (or sugar for sensitive skin). Add a couple of drops of essential oil for extra therapeutic properties (rose for dry skin, neroli to replenish cells).

Bridal spas

*Before you plunge into marital bliss, take a fabulous
dip in the pool at one of these luxury boltholes*

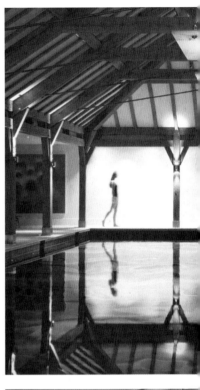

Your wedding day will be a flawless progression of sentiment and serenity – but right now, your best friends say they're 'definitely coming' but won't actually RSVP; your florist's gone AWOL and so has the vicar. You can't decide between Cabernet Sauvignon and Côtes du Rhône and you want to strangle your mother-in-law. But fear not, relaxation is at hand. You can banish stress, regain your inner peace – and buff your body – with a visit to one of these stunning spas.

Best for... getting some 'me time'

RAGDALE HALL
WHERE? Leicestershire
The perfect destination to kick-start your fitness levels and enjoy a spot of relaxation. Ragdale offers a fun, innovative programme of group workout classes, outside activities such as cycling, tennis, country hikes and Ragdale Express running sessions, plus four types of Aqua classes. If that's not enough, you can also have one-to-one personal training sessions and lifestyle and nutritional analysis. When the hard work and exertion is over, you can

unwind in Ragdale's renowned Thermal Spa, which has 12 luxurious heat and water experiences, which include the thunderous Cave Shower, heavenly Candle Pool and tranquil Waterfall. If all that doesn't leave you feeling like a new woman, the vast treatment menu will; ragdalehall.co.uk.

SPA INTERCONTINENTAL, PARK LANE
WHERE? London
This stunning day spa offers the ultimate is pre-wedding preparation and pampering. Treatment packages (think fabulous facials, blissful body wraps and floats, and relaxation therapies such as reflexology and hot stone massage) are available depending on your needs and budget, but all are guaranteed to give any bride-to-be the complete 'princess' experience. If you visit in the week before your big day, you can indulge in an OPI manicure and pedicure, BeauBronz natural spray tan and restorative GHD hair treatment; spaintercontinental.com.

GRAYSHOTT HALL
WHERE? Surrey
With its philosophy of 'health through inspiration, not deprivation' this spa offers specialist detox and cleansing programmes that can help you kick-start

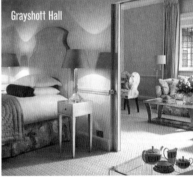

Grayshott Hall

weight loss, address sleeping issues and recharge your batteries while staying in beautiful country house surroundings. As well as a wide range of beauty and body treatments, Grayshott specialises in natural therapies including acupuncture, cranial osteopathy and the Alexander technique. Separate male and female spa areas house heat treatments, relaxation rooms and a hydrotherapy suite; grayshottspa.com.

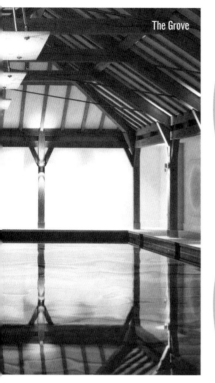

The Grove

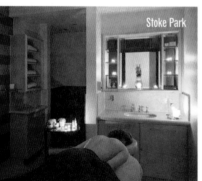

Stoke Park

Best for... bonding with your partner

ELEMIS DAY-SPA IN MAYFAIR
WHERE? **London**
Indulge in an exotic 45-minute Rasul for Two steam and mud treatment at London's first ever two-seater Rasul.

Perfect for couples to relax and detoxify, three different cleansing muds are applied to your face and body before you sit back and gently inhale the pure herb infused steam in your private chamber, then wash away the muds (and every last bit of tension) under a warm tropical rain shower. Also available is the Time for Two Couples Ritual, which includes an Exotic Frangipani Body Nourish Float and your choice of Skin Booster Facial or Well-Being Back Massage; timetospa.co.uk

SEQUOIA AT THE GROVE
WHERE? **Hertfordshire**
This 'groovy' grand country house spa hotel is as stylish as they come. With sumptuous, sexy bedrooms and suites, it's the perfect setting for a romantic weekend. The sleek spa has a black mosaic pool and cocoon-like relaxation room with velvet loungers, while the treatment menu offers holistic therapies

and ESPA ayurvedic treatments including a four-handed massage. For the ultimate pampering time together, treat yourself to a private spa session in the Couple's Suite, with deep, king-size bath, steam shower and two treatment beds for tandem relaxation; thegrove.co.uk.

HOAR CROSS HALL SPA RESORT
WHERE? **Staffordshire**
This elegant stately home is hidden away in 100 acres of countryside with lakes, formal gardens and even an Italian roof terrace. The spa's array of treatments is just as sumptuous, and you can now enjoy pampering with your partner in the double treatment room (we love the Cocooning Warm Oil Wrap). Holistic therapies include crystal healing, Indian head massages and reiki. And there's also golf, tennis, croquet, boules and archery on hand to keep non-spa loving partners happy; hoarcross.co.uk.

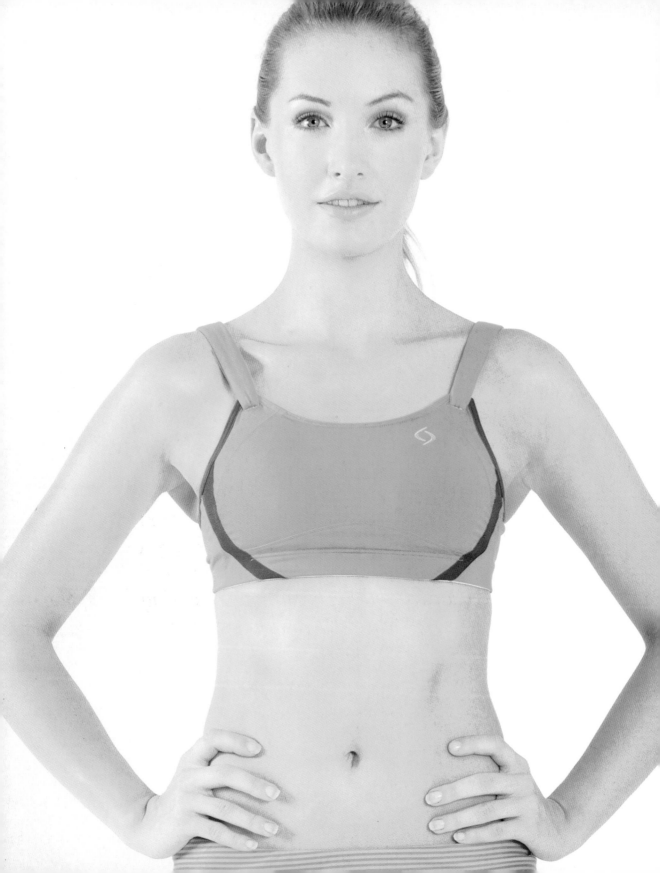

The workouts

Are you ready to sculpt your perfect bride's body? In this chapter you'll find a speedy total-body toning workout, to help you burn calories and blast fat. And there are another six workouts to target your trouble zones – banishing bingo wings, muffin top, bridesmaid's bulge and saddlebags. You don't even need a gym – you can do these sessions at home. There's also a six-week training plan to keep you motivated, plus a progress chart, so you can be sure you're staying on track with your efforts. Let's get sweaty!

How to use the WORKOUTS

With seven workouts to choose from, you can target your exercise sessions to meet your individual goals, from boosting your metabolism to sculpting your limbs

When it comes to shaping up for your wedding, time is of the essence. Not only do you have a deadline looming over you to reach your toning goals and target weight, but you also have to juggle a multitude of wedding-related appointments on top of your usual commitments. Ironically, you've probably got the most motivation you've ever had to exercise, and almost zero-time to fit it in.

Luckily, the key to achieving your goals is quality, not quantity, and over the following pages, you'll discover lots of multi-tasking moves that work together to create a time-saving, calorie-blitzing and body-sculpting exercise regime that will have you looking like the super-buff bride you've always wanted to be.

There are seven plans to choose from: a main workout that challenges your entire body to burn fat and tone every muscle, plus six, shorter, target workouts designed to offer extra toning on any trouble spots, such as arms or stomach. The beauty of this method is that you can mix them up according to your needs.

THE WARM-UP

Every workout you do, whatever type or however long – must start with a good warm-up. Do not skip it – a warm-up is essential to your training success and to help prevent injury. A warm-up increases the mobility of your major joints, helps your muscles and ligaments become more elastic and supple, and raises your pulse and core temperature which, in turn, increases blood flow so more oxygen can be pumped to your muscles

{ *'Luckily, the key to achieving your goals is quality, not quantity'* }

to make them work more effectively. Omitting warm-ups or not doing them properly can affect your training performance and contribute to small niggles and strains that might add up to serious injury over time – a definite no-no

if you want to get in the best shape of your life or avoid hobbling down the aisle. If you ever think about skipping a warm-up, take a moment to liken your muscles to a piece toffee: when toffee is cold, is it rock hard and liable to snap under pressure, just as muscle can. But when it's warm, it's much more pliable and less likely to break.

Find out how to warm up correctly on page 84.

THE MAIN WORKOUT

The main workout consists of eight exercises. That might not sound like many right now, but the exercises are designed to work many muscles of your body simultaneously, so you save lots of time compared to working muscle groups individually. Apart from shaving precious minutes from your workouts, there are many other benefits to be had from training multiple muscles in one go. The more muscles you use, the more challenging the exercises become, which then raises your heart rate and helps burn even more calories to melt fat and reveal muscle definition. Doing full-body moves that train your legs, bottom, core,

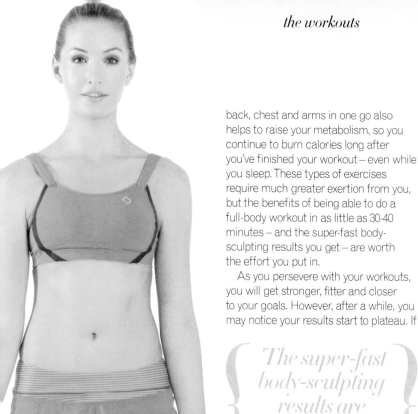

back, chest and arms in one go also helps to raise your metabolism, so you continue to burn calories long after you've finished your workout – even while you sleep. These types of exercises require much greater exertion from you, but the benefits of being able to do a full-body workout in as little as 30-40 minutes – and the super-fast body-sculpting results you get – are worth the effort you put in.

As you persevere with your workouts, you will get stronger, fitter and closer to your goals. However, after a while, you may notice your results start to plateau. If

> *'The super-fast body-sculpting results are worth the effort you put in'*

this happens, it's time to take your regime up a gear, either by increasing the weight of your dumbbells by 2.5kg, by performing an extra set of each exercise or by advancing to the exercise progressions offered for each move. You may find the progressions tough as many of them recruit more muscles than before, but they'll take your results to the next level.

THE TARGET WORKOUTS

The six Target workouts focus on key areas of your body to aid your bridal transformation: Arms & chest; Shoulders; Back; Abs & waist; Bottom and Legs. You might find you don't need to use the Target workouts at all and that the Main workout covers all your toning needs. But if you have real trouble zones – such as a jelly belly or wobbly saddle bags – you won't want them to be

seen when you're in a bikini on your honeymoon. Likewise, if you're concerned about your arms, shoulders and back being on show all day at your wedding, the Target workouts are where you can find additional moves to work those specific areas even more. While it's true you can't 'spot reduce' a particular area of the body, you can develop more lean muscle in a targeted area and improve its shape, especially when combined with a healthy diet and overall fat loss.

Each Target workout consists of three exercises to be performed in a circuit twice (perform one set of all three exercises, then repeat). There are many ways you can use the Target workouts to enhance your body-sculpting results. First, you can follow the six-week workout plan on page 122, which includes both Target zone and Main workouts. So for example, on a Target workout day, you'll warm up, then perform up to a maximum of three Target workouts for different body areas, followed by a cool-down.

Second, if you're feeling energetic or have good fitness levels, you can do a maximum of three Target workouts at the end of your Main workout, followed by a cool-down. And lastly, if you only have 15 minutes spare in your day, but want to do some kind of exercise, you can do just one Target workout for the area you're most concerned about, remembering to warm up before and cool down afterwards.

THE COOL-DOWN

We can't emphasise enough the importance of a cool-down, to encourage your body to return to its pre-exercise state and help keep muscles long and lean. Turn to page 120 to find out why a cool-down is so important to your training success, and discover the best stretches to perform.

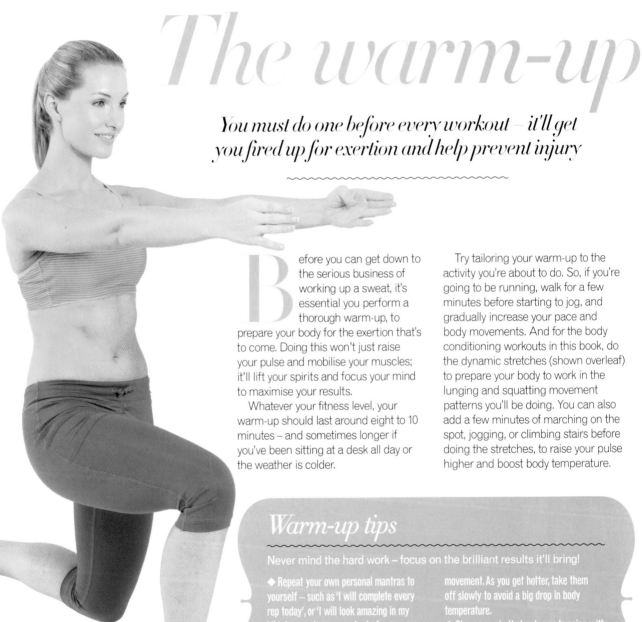

The warm-up

You must do one before every workout – it'll get you fired up for exertion and help prevent injury

Before you can get down to the serious business of working up a sweat, it's essential you perform a thorough warm-up, to prepare your body for the exertion that's to come. Doing this won't just raise your pulse and mobilise your muscles; it'll lift your spirits and focus your mind to maximise your results.

Whatever your fitness level, your warm-up should last around eight to 10 minutes – and sometimes longer if you've been sitting at a desk all day or the weather is colder.

Try tailoring your warm-up to the activity you're about to do. So, if you're going to be running, walk for a few minutes before starting to jog, and gradually increase your pace and body movements. And for the body conditioning workouts in this book, do the dynamic stretches (shown overleaf) to prepare your body to work in the lunging and squatting movement patterns you'll be doing. You can also add a few minutes of marching on the spot, jogging, or climbing stairs before doing the stretches, to raise your pulse higher and boost body temperature.

Warm-up tips

Never mind the hard work – focus on the brilliant results it'll bring!

◆ Repeat your own personal mantras to yourself – such as 'I will complete every rep today', or 'I will look amazing in my bikini on my honeymoon' – to focus your mind on what you want to achieve in the workout ahead.
◆ Wear layers during your warm-up to help retain the body heat you create through

movement. As you get hotter, take them off slowly to avoid a big drop in body temperature.
◆ Choose music that gets you buzzing with energy and feeling uplifted. It doesn't matter whether it's mellow or upbeat, as long as it triggers positive vibes that get you in the training zone.

CLOTHING: Moving Comfort Bra (movingcomfort.com); Studio2 leggings (dwsports.co.uk) Asics trainers (asics.co.uk)

YOUR DYNAMIC WARM-UP

These complementary moves will raise your pulse and get your muscles ready for action

SQUAT WITH OVERHEAD ARM SWING

Bend at the knees and hips to squat down and backwards, while simultaneously swinging your arms behind you (A). Return to standing, swinging your arms up and stretch overhead (B), to warm up your lower body, shoulders and back. Repeat for eight repetitions, starting off small and making your movements bigger as you continue. Keep your core engaged and chest lifted.

LUNGE WITH ROTATION

Standing upright with feet hip-width apart (A), lunge forwards, then rotate your torso to the same side as the lunging front leg (B). Make sure your leading knee does not go over the toe. Do eight repetitions on each leg, making the moves bigger with each one to wake up your legs, glutes, abs and spine.

ANGEL HUGS

Stand with your knees soft and core engaged. Open your arms out wide, gently pulling them backwards (A), then swing them to close around your body as if giving yourself a hug (B). Continue for eight reps, starting off small and getting bigger as you progress, to warm up your chest and back.

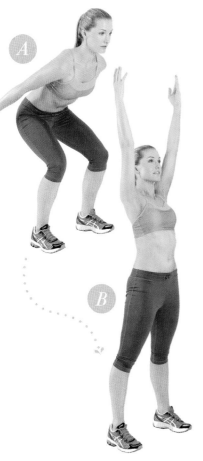

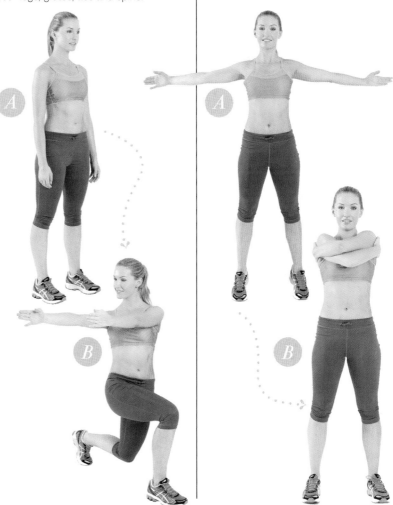

The workout

These exercises will get you to your wedding day with a sculpted and toned physique - we're talking wow factor!

LUNGE

WHY Works your hamstrings, quadriceps, and glutes for a shapely lower body.
HOW Stand with feet hip-width apart, hands on hips (A). With chest and chin high, inhale and take a long step forward with your left leg, until both knees are at 90° (B). Ensure your front knee doesn't go over your toes. Exhale, push off your left leg and return to start position. Do two sets of 12-15 reps on each side.
FOCUS on lowering down on your rear leg, to intensely work your bottom.

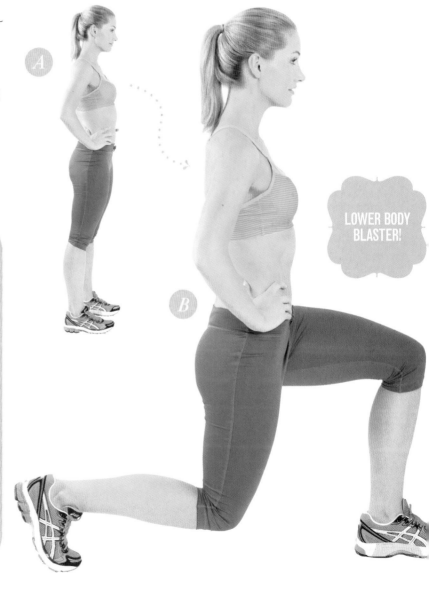

LOWER BODY BLASTER!

Progression
DISCO LUNGE

WHY Tones your lower body and upper back, for great posture.
HOW With hands by your sides (A), inhale and lunge while raising your arms. Keep your arms straight (B). Exhale, and lower your arms as you return to the start. Perform two sets of 12-15 reps on each side.
FOCUS on keeping your chest up, and core engaged.

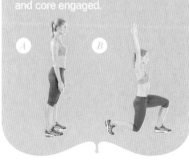

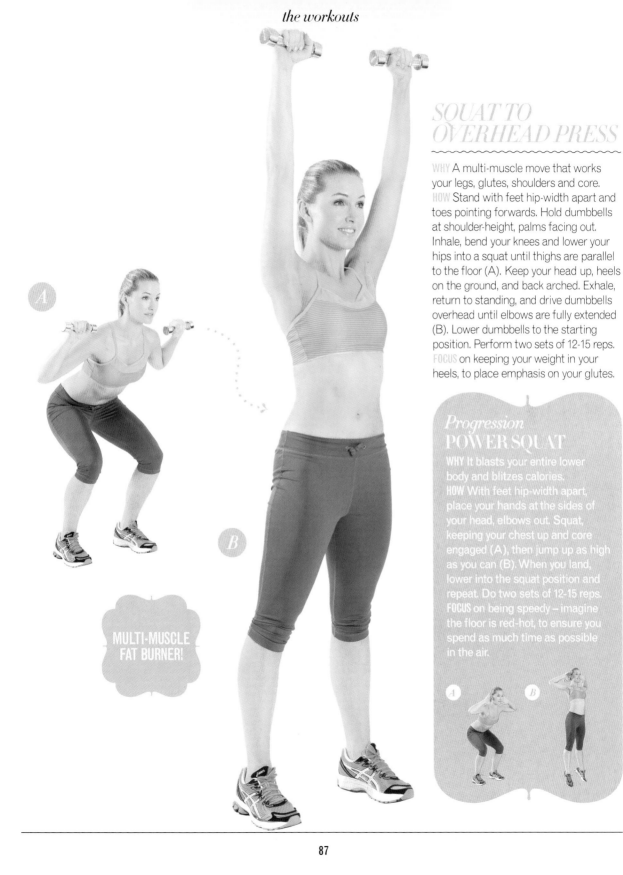

SQUAT TO OVERHEAD PRESS

WHY A multi-muscle move that works your legs, glutes, shoulders and core.
HOW Stand with feet hip-width apart and toes pointing forwards. Hold dumbbells at shoulder-height, palms facing out. Inhale, bend your knees and lower your hips into a squat until thighs are parallel to the floor (A). Keep your head up, heels on the ground, and back arched. Exhale, return to standing, and drive dumbbells overhead until elbows are fully extended (B). Lower dumbbells to the starting position. Perform two sets of 12-15 reps. FOCUS on keeping your weight in your heels, to place emphasis on your glutes.

Progression POWER SQUAT

WHY It blasts your entire lower body and blitzes calories.
HOW With feet hip-width apart, place your hands at the sides of your head, elbows out. Squat, keeping your chest up and core engaged (A), then jump up as high as you can (B). When you land, lower into the squat position and repeat. Do two sets of 12-15 reps. FOCUS on being speedy – imagine the floor is red-hot, to ensure you spend as much time as possible in the air.

MULTI-MUSCLE FAT BURNER!

WINDMILL

WHY Targets your core and waist for a sleek and sexy midriff.

HOW Hold your right arm above your head. Turn your left foot out, unlock your knees and look at your right hand (A). Exhale and lean to the left, sliding your left hand down your leg. right arm straight, strong and pointing up (B). Inhale, and return to standing. Do two sets of 12-15 reps on each side.

FOCUS on your breathing and engaging your core muscles throughout.

Progression
FLYING EAGLE TWIST

WHY The added weight doubles your effort and slims your waist.

HOW Stand with feet wide apart, toes pointing out, holding a dumbbell in your right hand above your head (A). Keeping the position of your right arm fixed, exhale and lower the body forward at the hips, twisting your torso to the right until your left hand touches the floor if you can do it (B). Inhale and stand up. Do two sets of 12-15 reps on each side.

FOCUS on keeping your core engaged throughout.

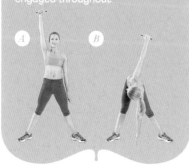

WHITTLES YOUR WAIST!

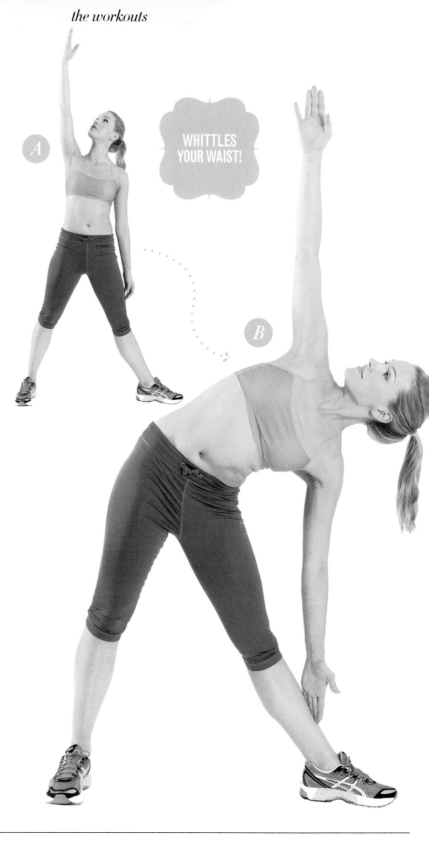

SIDE LUNGE

WHY Works your glutes, hamstrings, quads and thighs for ultra-toned legs.
HOW Stand with feet hip-width apart and hands on hips (A). Keeping your gaze forward and core engaged, inhale, take a big step to the left and bend your left knee to 90°. Keep your right leg straight (B). Exhale, push through the heel of your left foot and return to standing. Do two sets of 12-15 reps on both sides.
FOCUS on recruiting your inner-thigh muscles, especially when drawing your legs together to stand upright.

Progression
SIDE LUNGE WITH WOOD CHOP

WHY The added rotation blasts belly fat.
HOW With feet hip-width apart, hold one end of a dumbbell to your right ear (A). Inhale, lunge to the left while straightening your arms and arcing the dumbbell until it reaches the outside of your left ankle (B). Exhale, and raise your arms back to the start as you push off on your left foot to stand. Do two sets of 12-15 reps each side.
FOCUS on keeping your abs tight to work core and oblique muscles.

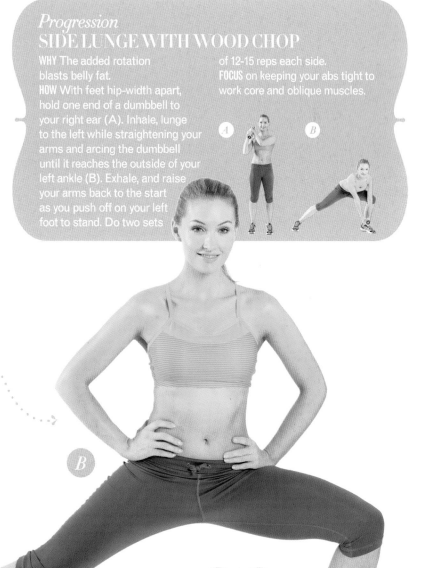

FOR TONED LEGS THAT LOOK GREAT IN HEELS

STIFF-LEGGED DEAD LIFT

WHY Works your hamstrings and glutes, to lift and tone your bottom.

HOW Standing feet hip-width apart, hold dumbbells with palms facing in (A). Keep your knees straight and core tight. Inhale, slowly bend forward from the hips and lower dumbbells until you feel an intense stretch in your hamstrings (B). Exhale, and reverse the direction, contracting your glutes as you rise upwards to the start position. Do two sets of 12-15 reps.

FOCUS on pushing your bottom backwards as you lower down to increase glutes activation.

Progression SINGLE-LEG DEAD LIFT

WHY Challenges your bottom and legs, for a delectable derrière.

HOW With a dumbbell in each hand, raise your right leg (A). Inhale, bend forward, lowering your torso until almost parallel to the floor. Extend your right leg (B). Keep a flat back. Pause, exhale, thrust your hips forward, and raise your torso back to the start.

FOCUS on engaging your core to maintain balance and use your glutes to control the movement.

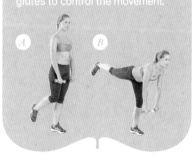

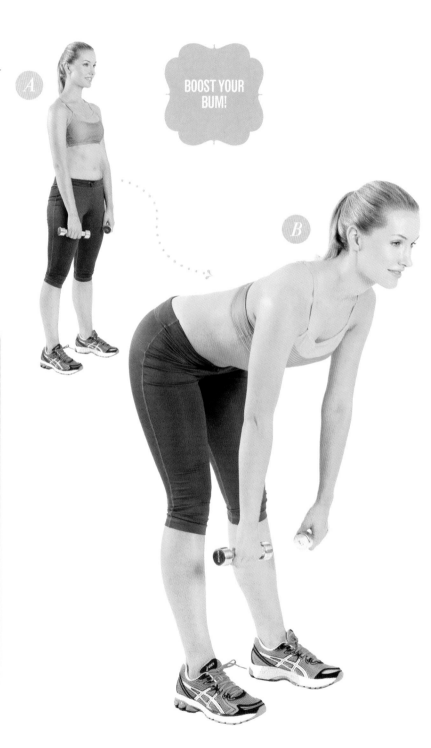

BOOST YOUR BUM!

WALKOUT

WHY Challenges your shoulders, arms, chest and core for upper-body toning.
HOW Stand with feet together and legs straight, keeping a slight bend in the knees. Bend forwards and place your hands on the ground in front of your feet (A). Slowly walk your hands forward one at a time (B), until you're in a full plank position (C). Slowly walk your hands back to starting the position. Do two sets of 12-15 reps.
FOCUS on engaging your core, to support the lower back and work your abs.

Progression WALKOUT WITH JUMP

WHY Adding an explosive jump will obliterate extra pounds.
HOW Perform the walkout as before. When you return to the starting position, bend at the knees (A), and power through your thighs to spring upwards and jump, lifting your arms above your head (B). Once you've landed, continue into the walkout exercise. Do two sets of 12-15 reps.

FOCUS on pulling your abs in throughout, and aim to land on the balls of your feet.

FOR SCULPTED SHOULDERS AND ARMS

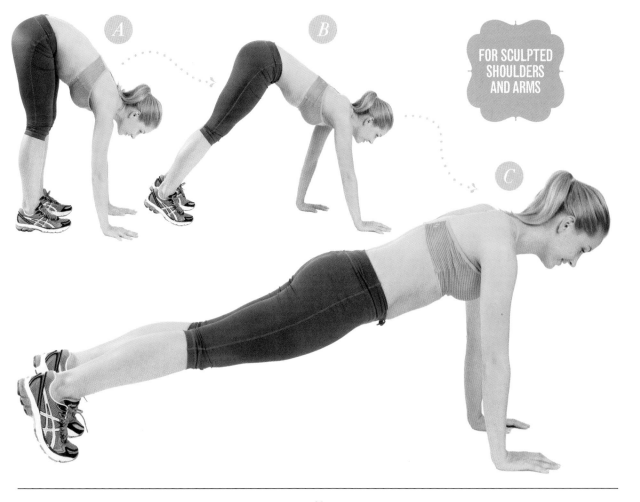

STRAIGHT-ARM PLANK

WHY This isolation exercise trains your deep core muscles for a flat stomach.
HOW Lie on the floor with hands beneath your shoulders. Contract your core and lift your body up so your weight is on your hands and toes. Keep your back straight so your body forms a straight line from neck to heels. Do not drop the hips (A). Hold this position for as long as you can or until technique starts to fail, building up from 30 seconds to one minute.
FOCUS on pulling your stomach muscles in tightly to protect your lower back.

Progression
SINGLE-LEG PLANK FLEX AND EXTEND

WHY Tones the whole body.
HOW Get into the straight-arm plank position. Lift your right leg off the floor. Contract your abs, round your back, lower your head and pull your right knee towards your face (A). Keeping the core, arms and legs strong, straighten your right leg out behind and lower your hips toward the floor without letting hips or legs touch the ground (B). Slowly pull your right knee back in. Build up to two sets of 12-15 reps on both sides.
FOCUS on extending your back to work your deep core muscles.

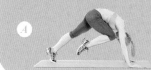

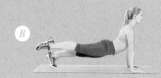

BUILDS GREAT BODY STRENGTH

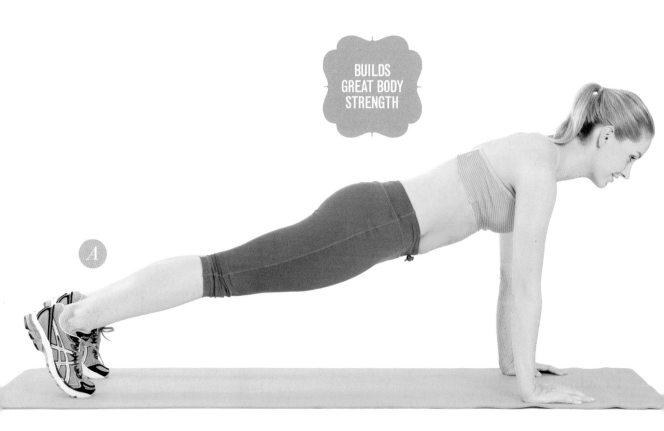

SIDE PLANK

WHY Strengthens your core for a neat, trim waist.

HOW Lie on your right side with your legs straight and feet stacked on top of each other. Place your right elbow under your right shoulder with your forearm out in front of you. Engage your core, lift your hips off the floor, and keep your body in a straight line from shoulders to ankles (A). Aim to hold for 30 seconds on each side, increasing to a minute as you progress.

FOCUS on keeping your body rigid and not allowing any part of your body to drop.

Progression
SIDE PLANK WITH ROTATION

WHY Whittles your waist, burns fat.
HOW In a right-side plank position (A), brace your abs and reach your left hand toward the ceiling. Slowly tuck your left arm under your body and twist forward until your torso is almost parallel to the floor (B). Hold for a second, and then return to the start. Do two sets of 12-15 reps on each side.
FOCUS on reaching upwards and under as far as you can for maximum 'twisting', while keeping your body rigid.

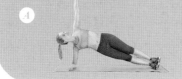

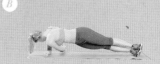

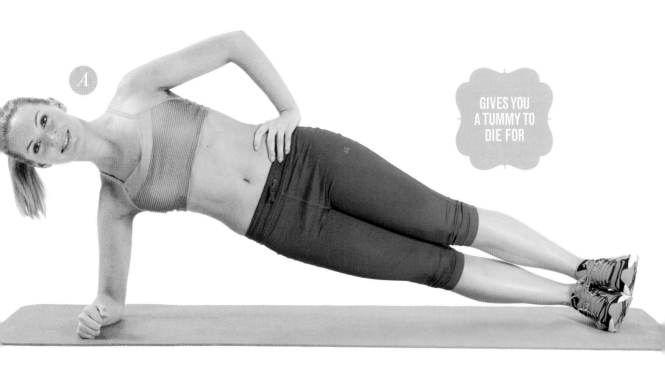

GIVES YOU A TUMMY TO DIE FOR

YOUR WORKOUT

1

LUNGE
PAGE 86

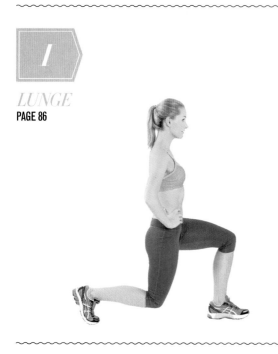

2

SQUAT TO OVERHEAD PRESS
PAGE 87

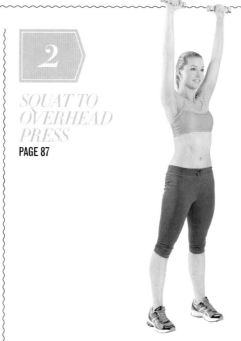

8

SIDE PLANK
PAGE 93

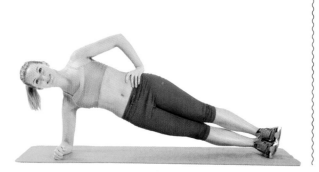

7

STRAIGHT-ARM PLANK
PAGE 92

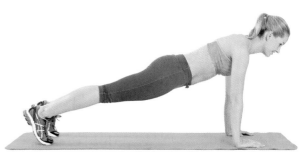

CIRCUIT

Now you've learnt the moves, this at-a-glance guide to your session will make it quicker and simpler

3

WINDMILL
PAGE 88

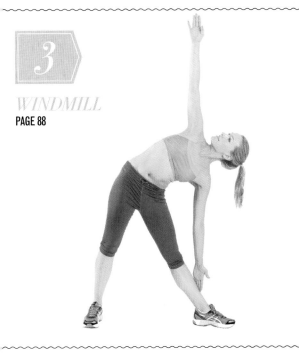

4

SIDE LUNGE
PAGE 89

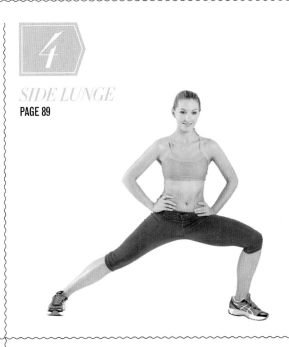

6

WALKOUT
PAGE 91

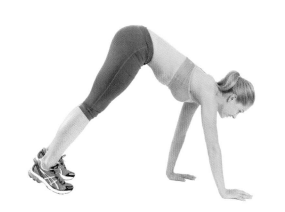

5

STIFF-LEGGED DEAD LIFT
PAGE 90

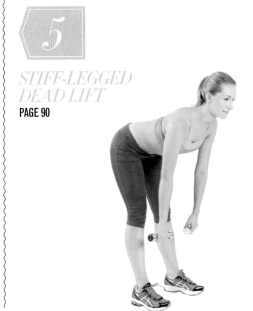

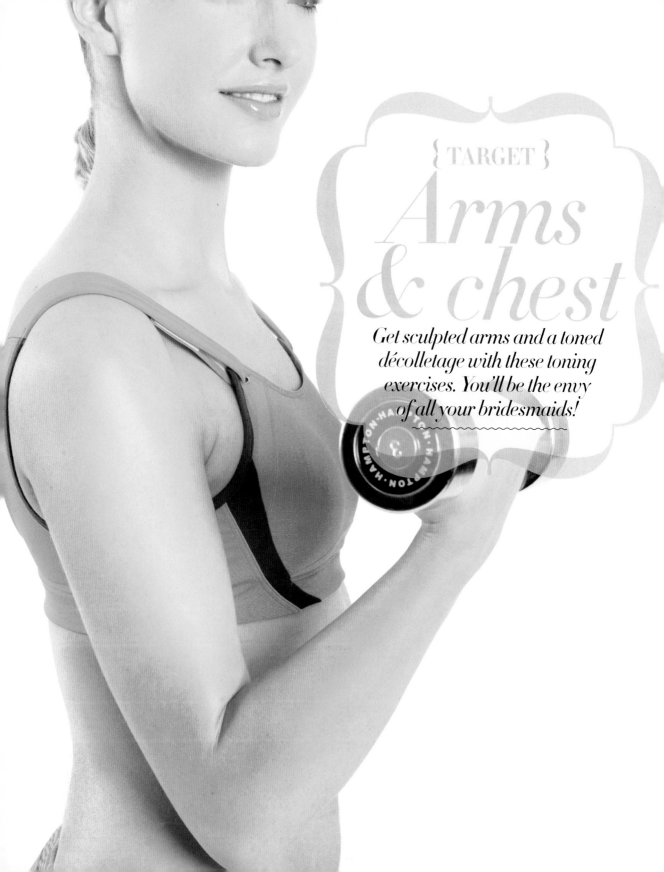

{ TARGET }

Arms & chest

Get sculpted arms and a toned décolletage with these toning exercises. You'll be the envy of all your bridesmaids!

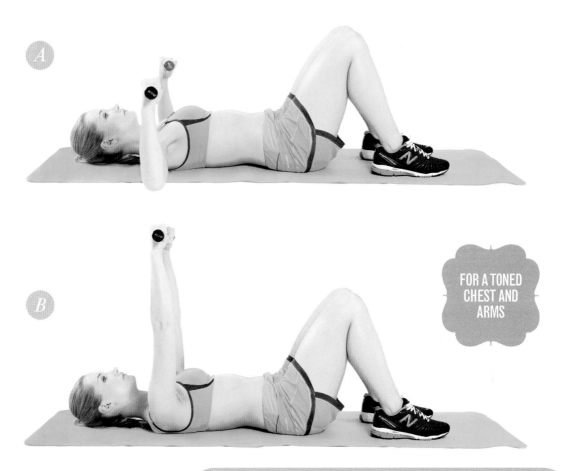

FOR A TONED CHEST AND ARMS

CHEST PRESS

WHY Works the pectoral muscles in the chest for a toned décolletage, and reduces the appearance of sagging skin.
HOW Lie on your back with your knees bent, feet flat on the floor. Hold dumbbells at shoulder level with your palms facing forwards and only your upper-arms on the floor (A). Exhale, and press the dumbbells up above your chest so they meet in the middle (B). Inhale, feel a contraction in your chest and slowly lower the dumbbells back down. Do two sets of 12-15 reps.
FOCUS on maintaining constant tension in your chest.

Progression
BRIDGE CHEST PRESS

WHY Adding a decline forces your chest to work harder and tones your core, glutes and hamstrings.
HOW Lie on your back, knees bent, and lift your hips off the floor so your body forms a straight line from knees to shoulders (A). Exhale, and press the dumbbells upwards (B). Inhale, and lower your upper arms to floor. Keep your hips lifted throughout. Do two sets of 12-15 reps.
FOCUS on your chest muscles as you push the dumbbells upwards, and keep your core and glutes tight.

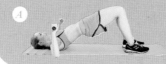

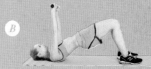

TRICEPS DIP

WHY Works the triceps muscles at the back of your arms to banish bingo wings.
HOW Sit on the edge of a chair with feet together. Place your palms to either side of your bottom. With your legs at 90°, bring your hips up and forwards off the chair (A). Inhale, and lower your body slowly until your arms form right angles (B). Exhale, and straighten your arms, raising your body back to the start. Do two sets of 12-15 reps.
FOCUS on using your triceps to return to the start, not your shoulders or legs.

Progression
TRICEPS DIP WITH EXTENDED LEGS

WHY The body weight on your triceps makes the move harder.
HOW Extend your legs so you're resting on your heels (A). Inhale, bend your arms to make a right angle while pointing your elbows behind you, and lower your hips (B). Exhale, and return to the start. Do two sets of 12-15 reps.
FOCUS on using your triceps muscles.

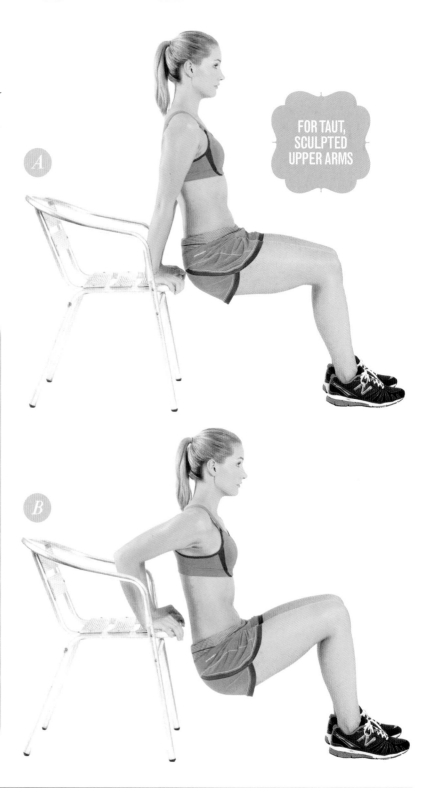

FOR TAUT, SCULPTED UPPER ARMS

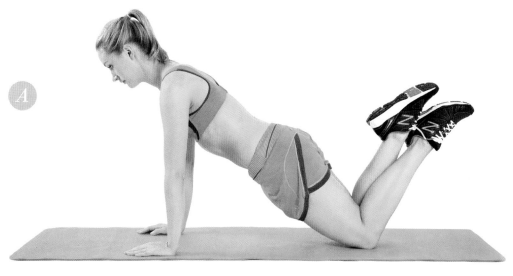

A

B

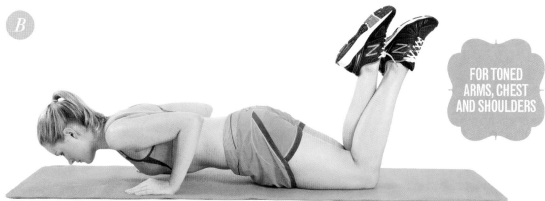

FOR TONED
ARMS, CHEST
AND SHOULDERS

3/4 PRESS-UP

WHY Works your upper body including your chest, triceps and core.
HOW Lie face-down with your hands on the floor at chest level, slightly wider than shoulder-width apart. Draw your belly button into your spine. Cross your feet and lift them off the floor. Exhale and push up with your hands (A). With your ears, shoulders and hips in line, inhale and lower back down so your arms are bent at 90 ° (B). Pause before you push back up to the start position. Perform two sets of 12-15 reps.
FOCUS on keeping your back flat by pulling your abs in tight throughout.

Progression
FULL PRESS-UP

WHY You increase the body weight placed on your upper body.
HOW Lie with your hands on the floor at chest level, slightly wider than shoulder-width apart. Brace your abs and push up until your arms are extended, so your body forms a straight line from your heels to your neck (A). Inhale, lower your body and pause, (B), then exhale and push yourself back to the start position (A). Perform two sets of 12-15 reps.
FOCUS on keeping your core engaged, to prevent your hips from dropping.

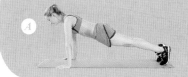

A

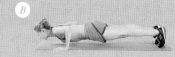

B

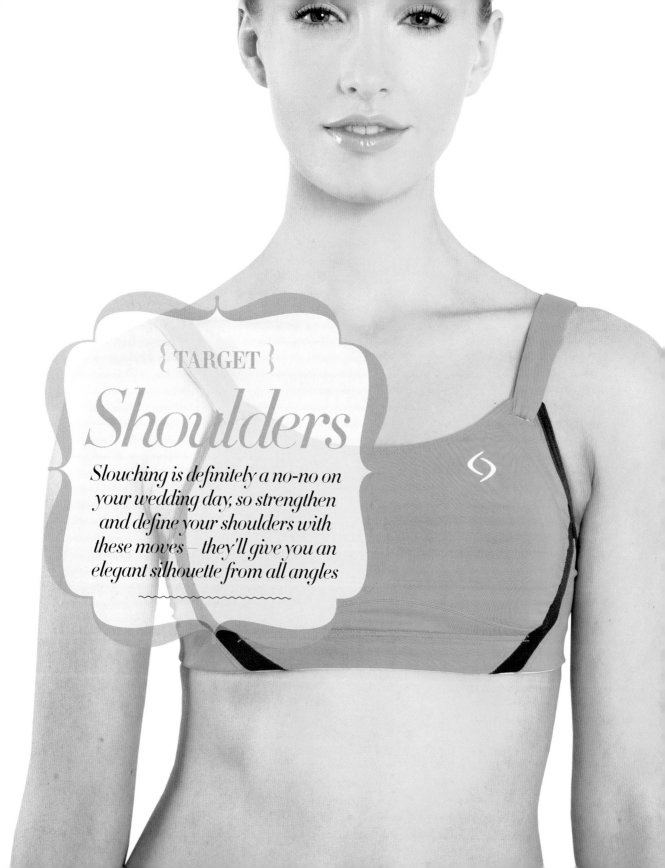

Shoulders

Slouching is definitely a no-no on your wedding day, so strengthen and define your shoulders with these moves – they'll give you an elegant silhouette from all angles

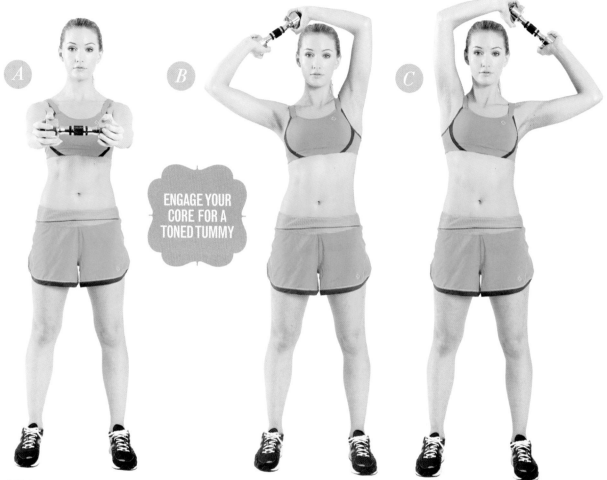

ENGAGE YOUR
CORE FOR A
TONED TUMMY

HALO

WHY It works your shoulders in
all directions.

HOW Stand holding a dumbbell in each
hand. Bend your knees slightly, with your
weight equally distributed through both
feet. Raise the dumbbell to chest level,
keeping your arms straight and core
strong (A). Bend your arms and move
the dumbbell behind your head in a
circular motion (B) and (C) until your
arms are back to the start position. Do
12-15 reps clockwise, then repeat in an
anti-clockwise direction. Do two sets.

FOCUS on a spot on the wall and
keep looking straight at it to help
maintain balance.

Progression
HALO ON ONE LEG

WHY You get the upper-body
benefits, and your core and legs
work hard to keep you stabilised.
HOW With your knees slightly bent,
raise one foot slightly off the floor
behind you. Brace your abs and
raise the dumbbell to chest level
with straight arms (A). Complete
12-15 reps of circling the dumbbell
around your head in a clockwise
direction as above (B), then
repeat in an anti-clockwise
direction (C). Do two sets.

FOCUS on keeping your abs pulled
in and moving in a slow and
controlled manner.

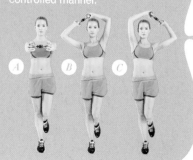

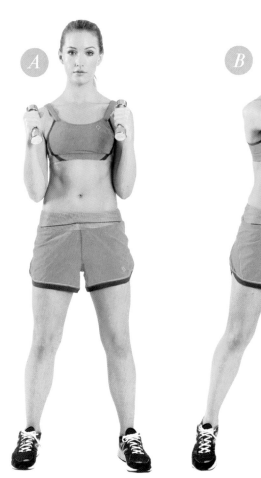

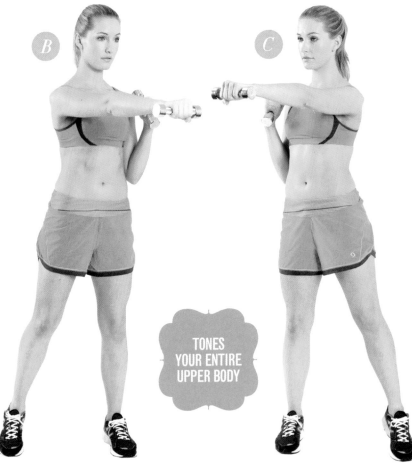

TONES YOUR ENTIRE UPPER BODY

DUMBBELL PUNCH

WHY Works every muscle in your shoulders, for amazing definition.
HOW Stand with feet hip-width apart and knees soft. Holding dumbbells, bend your elbows and raise them to shoulder height (A). Engage your abs, twist your torso to the left, and extend your right arm out, palm facing down (B). Return to the start position and repeat on the other side, twisting your torso to the right and extending your left arm (C). That's one rep. Do two sets of 12-15 reps.
FOCUS on keeping the movement controlled and not locking the elbows.

Progression
DUMBBELL PUNCH WITH UPPERCUT

WHY It works your upper body for total toning.
HOW Lower the dumbbells to hip-height with your elbows bent. Keeping your left hand at your hip, twist your torso to the left and 'punch' the right dumbbell upwards and across towards your left shoulder (A). Return the dumbbell to your hip, and repeat on the other side (B) for one rep. Alternate your arms as fast as possible. Do 12-15 reps.

FOCUS on keeping your abs tight throughout the exercise.

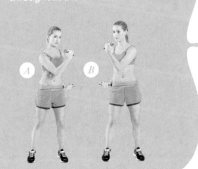

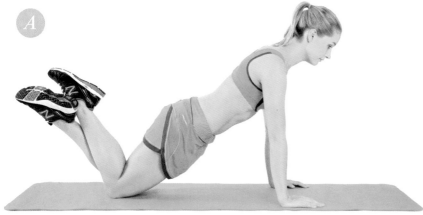

A

3/4 WALKING PLANK

WHY This double-whammy move sculpts your shoulders and strengthens the core.
HOW On your hands and knees, cross your feet, lift them off the floor and engage your core. Walk your hands forwards until your body is in a straight line from your knees to the neck (A). Lower your left forearm to the floor (B), then the right one, so you are in an elbow plank (C). Step your right hand back onto the mat, then the left, pushing yourself back up to the start position. Do one set of 12-15 reps leading with the left hand, and the second with the right.
FOCUS on keeping your torso immobile.

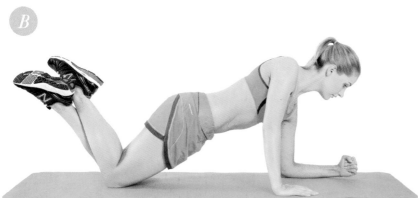

B

Progression
WALKING PLANK

WHY The increase in body weight from extending your legs will supercharge this exercise.
HOW Instead of supporting your body weight between your arms and knees, extend your legs fully behind you so your body weight is placed on your hands and toes (A). 'Walk' your arms down and up as before (B), doing two sets of 12-15 reps.
FOCUS on keeping your core strong, to prevent pressure on your back.

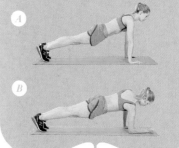

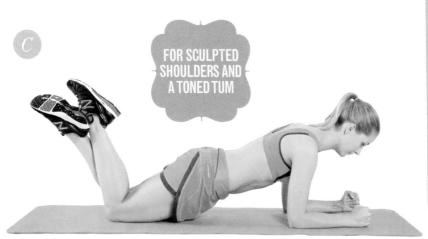

C

FOR SCULPTED SHOULDERS AND A TONED TUM

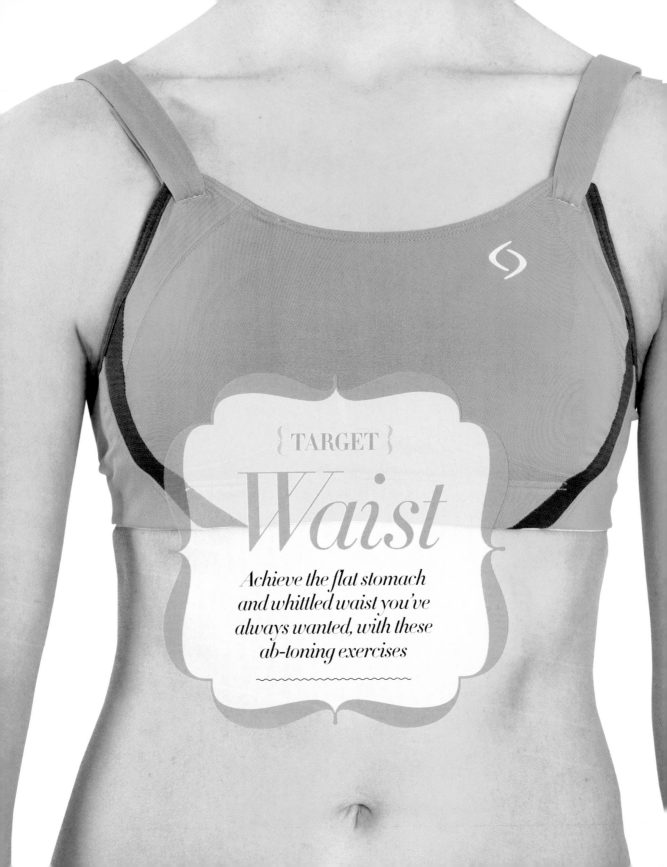

{ TARGET }

Waist

Achieve the flat stomach
and whittled waist you've
always wanted, with these
ab-toning exercises

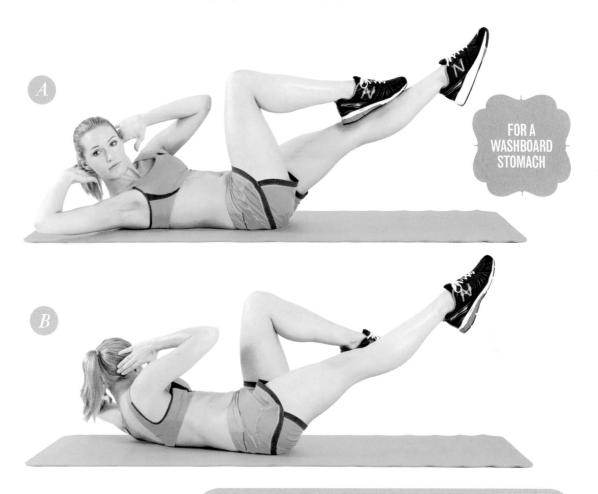

FOR A
WASHBOARD
STOMACH

BICYCLE CRISS-CROSS

WHY This twisting crunch works your core, upper and lower abs and obliques.
HOW Lie with your feet off the floor, knees up above your hips. Place your fingertips to your ears, keeping elbows wide, and lift your head off the floor. Exhale, peel your left shoulder across to your right side as you extend your left leg, bringing your left elbow to your right knee (A). Inhale, return to centre and exhale to go in the opposite direction to complete rep (B). Do two sets of 12-15 reps.
FOCUS on keeping your upper back off the floor, to maintain tension in your abs.

Progression
V-SIT CRISS-CROSS

WHY With more of your body weight to support, your abs work harder.
HOW Sit upright with your knees bent and feet flat on the floor. Brace your abs and lean back to 45°, holding your fingertips to your ears. Exhale, and bring your left elbow and right knee together, crunching diagonally across to the right and extending your left leg out (A). Inhale as you return to centre, and repeat on the other side to complete one rep (B). Do two sets of 12-15 reps.
FOCUS on balancing on your bottom and pulling in your abs.

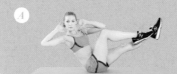

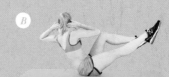

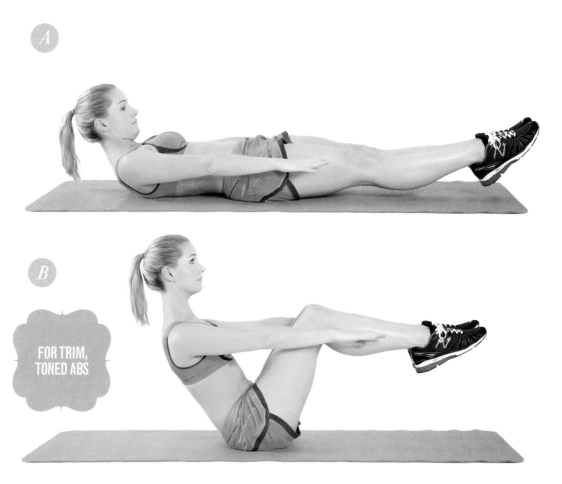

FOR TRIM,
TONED ABS

V-SIT

WHY Works your core and upper and lower abs for a super-flat stomach.
HOW Lie face up, hands by your sides and palms facing down. Contract your abs, lift your legs a few inches off the ground and peel your shoulders and arms off the floor (A). Exhale, and use your abs to sit up to 45°, while also pulling your knees towards your chest, so only your bottom remains on the floor (B). Inhale, and return to (A). Do two sets of 12-15 reps.
FOCUS on keeping your stomach pulled in, and avoid using momentum to pull your torso off the floor.

Progression JACKKNIFE

WHY With your limbs extended, you'll work your abs harder.
HOW Lie on the floor, feet flexed and hands extended behind (A). Contract your abs, exhale, and raise your upper body, bringing both legs towards your hands to touch your feet (B). Inhale as you lower your limbs but don't let them touch the floor, then raise again. Do two sets of 12-15 reps.
FOCUS on using your abs to lift your arms and legs off the floor; make controlled movements.

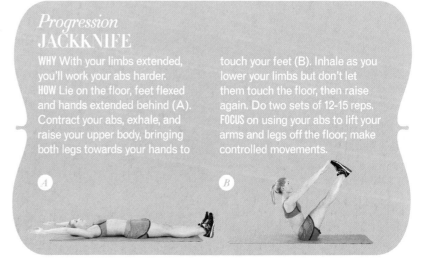

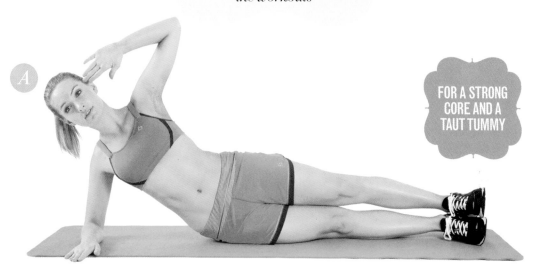

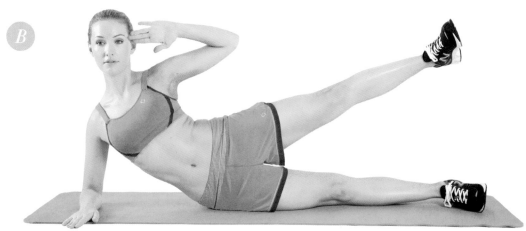

FOR A STRONG CORE AND A TAUT TUMMY

SIDE JACKKNIFE

WHY Targets your core and obliques (side abs) for a sexy, streamlined waist.

HOW Lie on your right side with your feet together. Hold your left fingertips to your ear and place your right forearm on the floor (A). Exhale, and simultaneously raise your torso and left leg into the air, so they come as close together as possible (B). Contract your oblique muscles, inhale, and slowly reverse the direction to return to the start position. Do two sets of 12-15 reps on each side.

FOCUS on preventing your torso from twisting, by imagining the back of your body is against a wall.

Progression
FULL EXTENSION SIDE JACKKNIFE

WHY It boosts your core stability.

HOW Kneel on the floor and lean over to your right, supporting yourself on your right hand. Extend your left leg and place your left hand on your ear, elbow upwards (A). Exhale, and raise your left foot to hip-height, while extending your left arm and crunching your waist (B). Inhale, and lower your limbs. Do two sets of 12-15 reps on each side.

FOCUS on controlling the move from your obliques and hips.

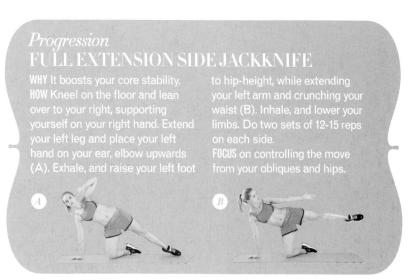

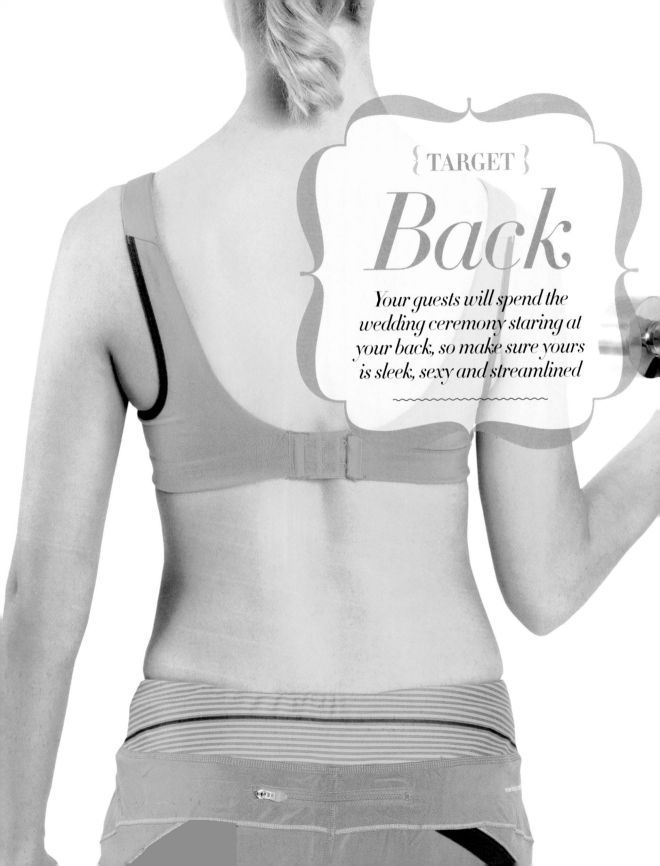

Back

Your guests will spend the wedding ceremony staring at your back, so make sure yours is sleek, sexy and streamlined

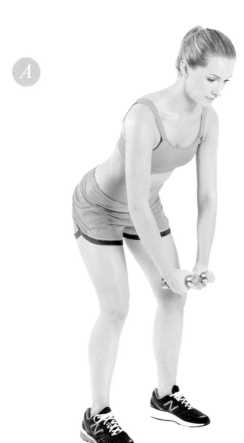

A

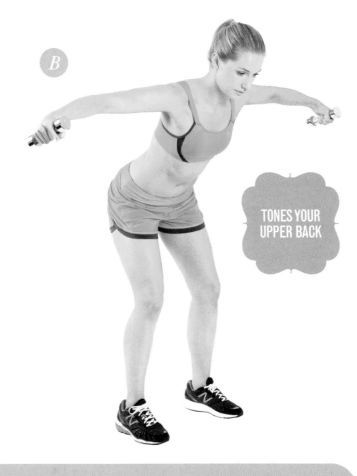

B

**TONES YOUR
UPPER BACK**

STANDING REVERSE FLYE

WHY Works your back and rear shoulders, to help you stand tall.

HOW Stand with your feet hip-width apart, knees slightly bent and hips hinged. Keeping your back flat and core engaged, hold two dumbbells in front of your thighs, a slight bend at the elbow, palms facing each other (A). Maintaining bent arms throughout, exhale and bring both arms up and out until your elbows are slightly higher than your shoulders (B). Inhale, and lower your arms back to the start. Do two sets of 12-15 reps.

FOCUS: on retracting and squeezing your shoulder blades together on each rep.

Progression
REVERSE FLYE WITH GLUTE EXTENSION

WHY Works your back, shoulders, core, glutes and hamstrings.

HOW With your right foot slightly behind your left, resting on your toes, hold the dumbbells at your sides, palms facing each other (A). Exhale and hinge forward from your hips, raising your right leg back until your torso and right leg are parallel to the floor. At the same time, raise your arms to shoulder-height, squeezing your shoulder blades together (B). Inhale, then return to the starting position. Do one set of 12-15 reps lifting your right leg, and a second set with the left.

FOCUS on using your glutes to lift and lower your extending leg.

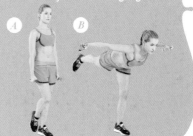

A

B

A

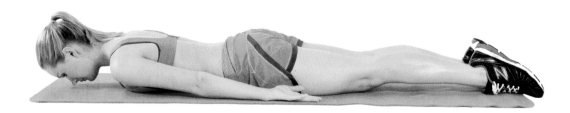

B

**GET A
STRONG CORE**

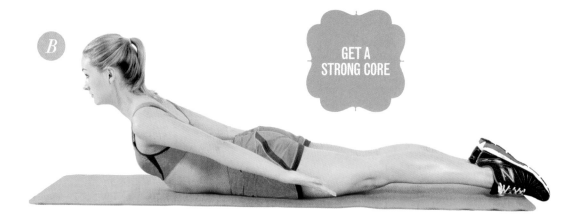

LOWER BACK EXTENSION

WHY Strengthens your back and core for a balanced torso.

HOW Lie face-down with your arms by your sides and forehead near the floor (A). Inhale and, as you exhale, lift your upper body off the floor, keeping your hips and legs rooted to the ground (B). Hold for a count of two, inhale, and slowly lower your torso back down. Do two sets of 12-15 reps.

FOCUS on lifting from your lower back muscles. Squeeze your glutes to stabilise your movement.

Progression
FULL BACK EXTENSION

WHY Works your back, core, glutes and hamstrings to the max.

HOW Lie face down with your arms straight, extended forwards, and head and neck in a neutral position (A). Keeping your midsection stable, inhale and, as you exhale, lift your arms and legs off the floor, feeling the contraction in your lower back and glutes (B). Hold for a count of two, inhale and slowly lower your limbs back down. Do two sets of 12-15 reps.

FOCUS on maintaining slow and controlled movements. Keep your gaze down and don't bob your head.

A

B

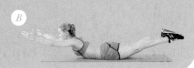

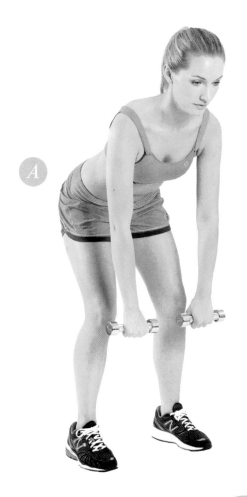

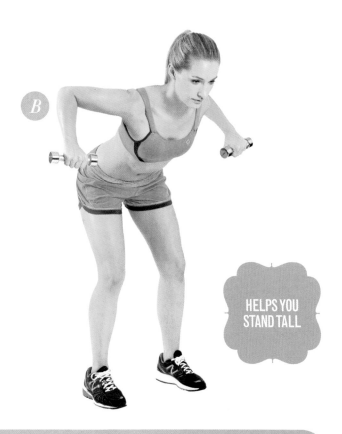

HELPS YOU STAND TALL

BENT-OVER ROW

WHY Works your upper back to prevent slouching and help you stand tall.
HOW Stand with your feet hip-width apart, and toes pointing forwards. Hold your dumbbells in front of you, palms facing your thighs. Bend your knees and lean forward at your hips, keeping your back straight (A). Raise the dumbbells to your chest, pulling your shoulder blades together in a 'rowing' action. Keep your elbows high (B). Lower the dumbbells to the start. Do two sets of 12-15 reps.
FOCUS on contracting the muscles in your upper back.

Progression
SINGLE-LEG DEADLIFT WITH ROW

WHY Works your back, shoulders, core and lower body.
HOW Standing with feet parallel, raise your right foot behind you. Holding a dumbbell in each hand with palms facing your thighs, exhale, hinge forward from your hips and raise your right leg back. At the same time, lower the dumbbells to the floor (A). 'Row' the dumbbells towards your chest (B), then lower your right leg and let the dumbbells return to your sides as you stand up. Do one set of 12-15 reps, raising your right leg, then repeat on the other side.
FOCUS on keeping your core tight.

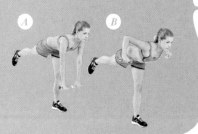

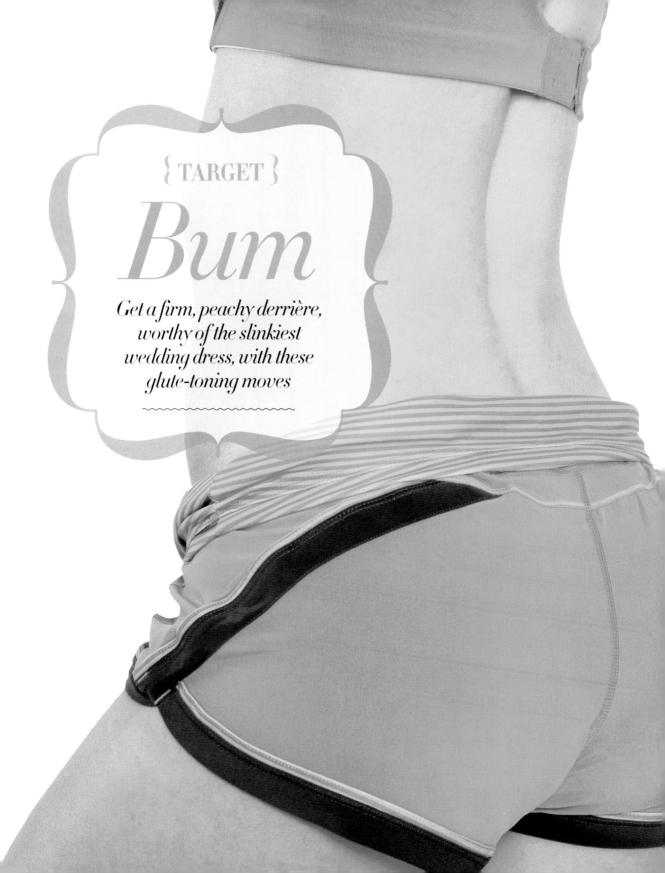

Bum

Get a firm, peachy derrière, worthy of the slinkiest wedding dress, with these glute-toning moves

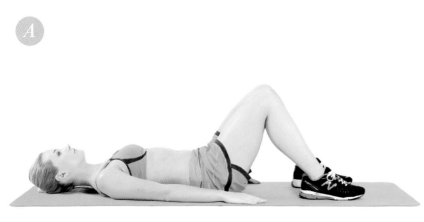

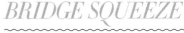

BRIDGE SQUEEZE

WHY Intensely targets your glutes, and recruits your thigh, core and lower-back muscles.

HOW Lie with your knees bent, feet flat on the floor and hands palms-down at your sides (A). Keeping your back straight, lift your hips off the floor and contract your glutes (B). Hold for 10 seconds, then pulse your hips down a few inches (C) and back up. Do 12-15 pulses for one set. Lower your body back to the floor, take a rest and repeat the set.

FOCUS on lengthening your legs from hip bones to knees. Don't arch your back.

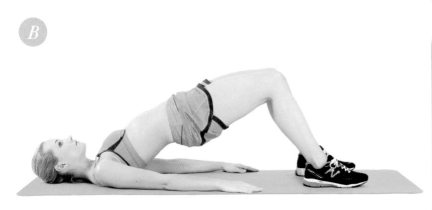

Progression
ONE-LEGGED BRIDGE SQUEEZE

WHY Works your glutes even harder.
HOW Lying on your back, legs bent and feet on the floor, brace your abs, straighten one leg and lift it off the floor, keeping your stomach flat (A). Raise your hips into bridge (B). Lower and raise your hips a few inches for 12-15 pulses. Lower and repeat on the other leg, rest and do a second set.
FOCUS on squeezing your glutes.

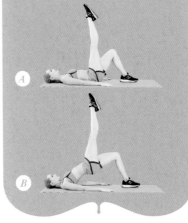

TONES YOUR BUM AND THIGHS

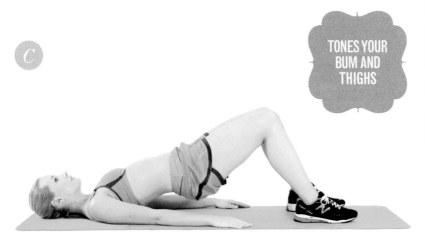

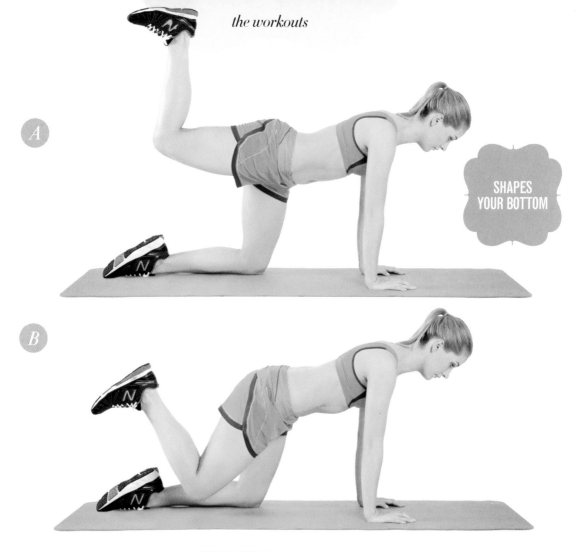

A

B

SHAPES
YOUR BOTTOM

DONKEY KICK

WHY Targets your hamstrings and glutes
to lift, tone and shape your bottom.
HOW Get on all fours with your hands
under your shoulders. Keeping your right
knee bent at 90°, flex your foot and lift
your leg until your thigh is parallel to
floor, squeezing your right glute (A).
Lower your leg back down, not letting
your knee touch the floor (B), then raise
again. Perform 12-15 reps. Next, raise
your leg to (A), and pulse it up and down
a few inches for 20 reps. Lower your leg
and repeat on the other side to do one
set. Rest, and do a second set.
FOCUS on lifting the leg as high as you can.

Progression
BOOTY BLASTERS

WHY Works the smaller muscles
at the sides of your glutes.
HOW From all fours, lift your right
leg straight out to your side,
keeping your foot flexed (A).
Lower your leg without letting your
foot touch the floor (B), then
contract your glutes to return to

position (A) and repeat 12-15
times. Quickly pulse your leg up
and down a few inches for 20 reps.
Repeat everything on the other
side. Rest, and repeat on both legs.
FOCUS on keeping your shoulders
and hips as square to the floor
as possible.

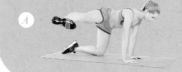

A

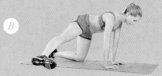

B

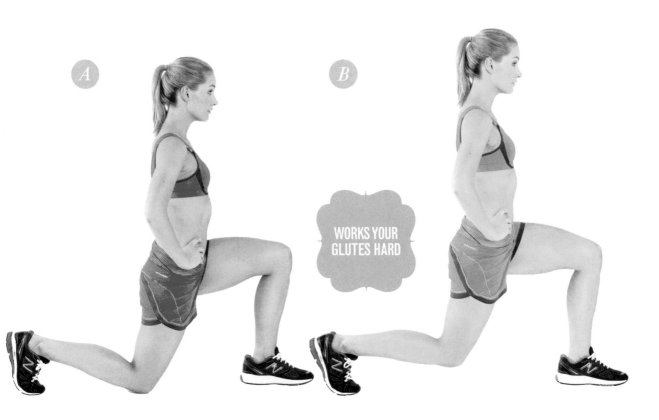

WORKS YOUR GLUTES HARD

LOW-AS-YOU-CAN-GO LUNGE

WHY These are super tough on your glutes, but promote a peachy posterior.
HOW Step your left leg forward into a lunge and, keeping your core engaged and chest lifted, lower your right knee to the floor (A). Lift your right knee half an inch off the ground and hold for 15 seconds (B). Then do 20 small 'bouncing' lunges, slowly rising up an inch off the ground then tapping your knee gently to the floor. Switch legs and repeat. Rest, then do a second set on both legs.
FOCUS on controlled bouncing.

Progression
LUNGE WITH DUMBBELLS

WHY Adding extra weight means your glutes have to work even harder to lift and lower.
HOW Do the low-as-you-can-go lunges as above, but this time holding either one or two dumbbells (A) and (B). You can also hold the pose for longer in the first phase of the exercise, or increase the number of bouncing lunges you do on each leg to increase the intensity.

FOCUS on using the back leg to power the 'up-and-down' movement, to tone your glutes rather than your thighs.

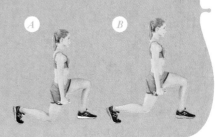

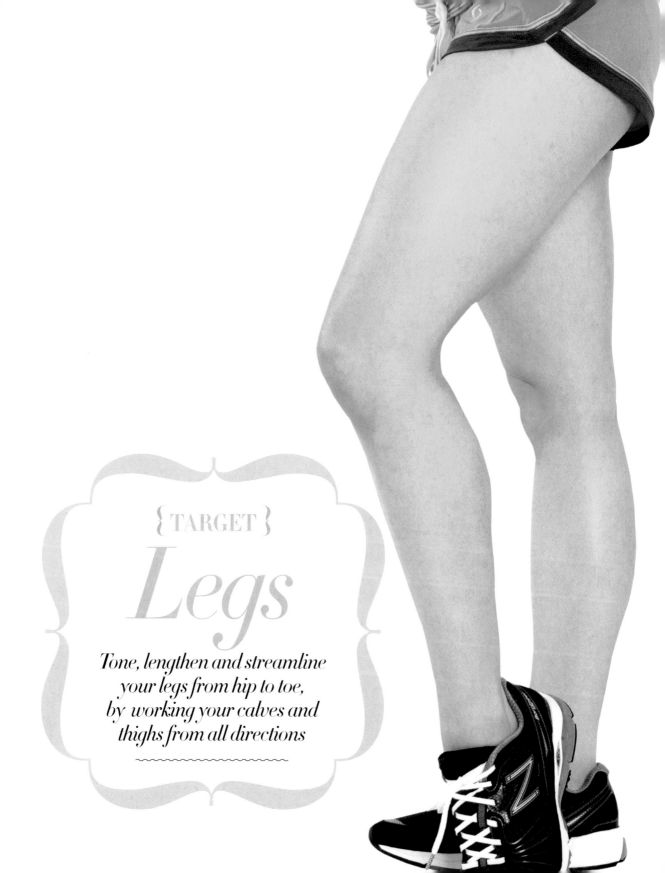

Legs

*Tone, lengthen and streamline
your legs from hip to toe,
by working your calves and
thighs from all directions*

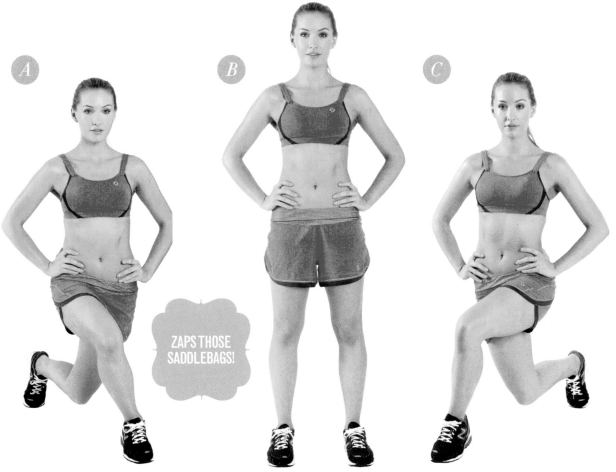

ZAPS THOSE
SADDLEBAGS!

CROSSOVER LUNGE

WHY Works the hamstrings, glutes, hips and inner and outer thighs to blast away saddlebags.

HOW Stand with your feet hip-width apart and hands on hips. Inhale, and step your right leg forward and diagonally across to the outside of your left leg while bending your knees to 90° (A). Exhale and return to the start position (B), then repeat by leading with your left leg and crossing over your right foot (C). Keep your chin and chest lifted throughout. Do two sets of 12-15 reps on both sides.

FOCUS on bending your back leg with control, to prevent your front toe going over your front knee.

Progression
CROSSOVER LUNGE WITH BICEP CURL

WHY The added weight increases the lower-body benefits and also tones your arms.

HOW Stand with your feet hip-width apart, a dumbbell in each hand and arms by your sides. Inhale and lunge diagonally forward, as above, while curling the dumbbells toward your shoulders (A). Exhale, return to standing and lower the dumbbells (B). Alternate your legs (C), doing two sets of 12-15 reps on each side.

FOCUS on engaging your core, keeping your shoulders back and down, arms close to your torso.

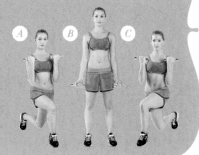

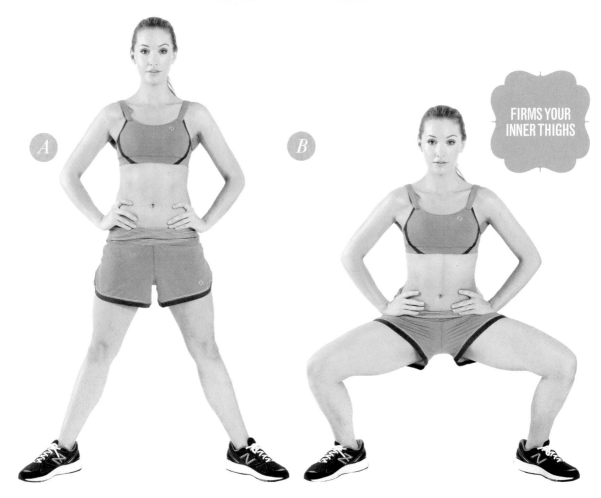

A

B

FIRMS YOUR INNER THIGHS

PLIÉ SQUAT

WHY This exercise is fantastic for toning your glutes and inner thighs.

HOW With your hands on your hips and feet wider than shoulder-width apart, turn your knees and toes out (A). Keeping your weight pressed into your heels, tuck your tailbone under and contract your glutes. Inhale and lower for a count of two (B). Pause, exhale, and return to the start position for a count of two while imagining you're wearing roller skates and using your inner thighs to help draw your legs back together. Do two sets of 12-15 reps.

FOCUS on engaging your inner thighs.

Progression
PLIÉ SQUAT WITH CALF RAISE

WHY This also works your calf muscles for total leg toning, from your hips to your ankles.
HOW From a plié squat (A), rise onto your toes and contract your calf muscles (B). This will place more emphasis on your inner thighs. Lower your heels and return to standing, knees straight. Perform two sets of 12-15 reps.
FOCUS on keeping your balance by making sure your core is fully engaged and focusing on an object in front of you, at about head height.

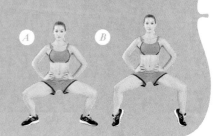

A   B

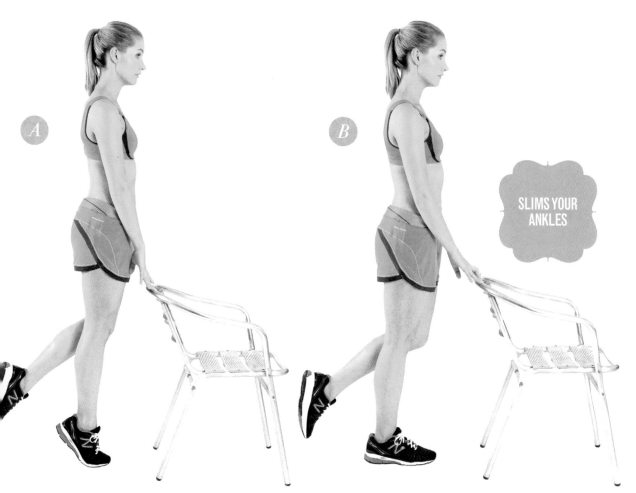

A

B

SLIMS YOUR
ANKLES

ONE-LEGGED CALF RAISE

WHY Say goodbye to fleshy ankles with this lower-leg toning move.

HOW Stand on your right foot, holding on to back of chair for balance. Raise your left leg bent behind you. Contract your calf muscles and raise your right heel off the floor to balance on tip toes (A). Hold for two seconds, then lower your heel back down to the floor (B). Do two sets of 12-15 reps on both sides.

FOCUS on rising up as high as possible onto your toes.

Progression
ONE-LEGGED CALF RAISE WITH SQUAT

WHY The added squat will work your legs even harder, toning the front of your thighs.

HOW Stand as above. Bend your right leg behind you, then rise up onto your toes (a), and lower your left knee so you lower into a single-leg squat (c). Return to standing, keeping your right leg off the ground throughout. Do two sets of 12-15 reps on both legs.

FOCUS on lifting the heel of your supporting leg and lowering as deeply as you can into the squat.

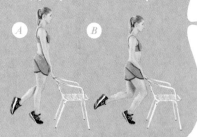

A

B

The cool-down

Ease out your muscles with these tried and tested moves

The cool-down phase of your workout is just as essential to your training success as the warm-up section, and should never be skipped – not even for a meeting with the vicar! Cooling down is vital, as it allows your body to come back to its pre-exercise state. This is particularly important after strenuous activity, when the blood that has been diverted to working muscles can 'pool' in your extremities, making you feel dizzy and nauseous if you suddenly stop exercising.

Stretching also keeps your muscles long and lean, improves posture, helps re-align your body, prevents injury and eases post-exercise muscle soreness. So don't be tempted to give it a miss.

HOW TO COOL DOWN

Firstly, it's important you keep moving. No matter how tired you feel, avoid the temptation to flop on the floor. Instead, spend a few minutes doing light activity that involves the muscle groups you've been using. If you've been running or walking, slowly reduce your pace and make your movements smaller until

> *'Don't be tempted to skip the cool-down – it's vital for your progress'*

your pulse is back to normal. If you've been doing strength training, try marching on the spot and raising your arms gently up and down to encourage blood to return back to your heart, reducing your movements gradually.

Once your breathing is back to normal, you can start to stretch out. Turn the page for some of the best cool-down stretches to use after your workout.

COOL-DOWN TIPS

Re-oxygenate your body by taking some deep breaths. Slowly breathe in for four counts and release, doing this several times while you cool down.

Have some layers ready to put on during your cool-down. This will prevent your core body temperature from dropping too quickly, and keep your muscles warm and pliable while you stretch.

Maintain existing suppleness by holding your stretches for 10-15 seconds. To develop flexibility, hold stretches for 10-15 seconds, relax until the tension has reduced, then stretch again for a further 10-15 seconds.

Chill out, take stock

Don't rush your cool down, or feel pressured to move on to the next thing in your day – enjoy the moments of calm!

◆ Apart from being physically beneficial, a good cool-down can help you relax, mentally unwind and take some time out from the stresses of planning your wedding. It also provides the perfect opportunity for you to reflect on what you've just achieved with your workout. While you're stretching, consider if certain exercises felt easier to do than in previous sessions – if you felt less out of breath, stronger or more supple – and be encouraged by the fitness and health gains you're making.

◆ Tune in to your emotions. Even if you feel exhausted, you should also feel proud of what you've accomplished, happy in the knowledge that every workout you do moves you closer to your ultimate goal. Remember, the more you associate your workouts with positive feelings, the more likely you are to stick to your programme in the long run – and reap even more benefits!

◆ Why not tune in to your favourite feelgood chillout tunes while you stretch? You're bound to finish on a high!

COOL-DOWN STRETCHES

Do each of these moves to ease out your whole body

 1 ### HAMSTRING STRETCH
Lie on the floor with your knees bent and feet flat. Raise one leg and grab it with both hands (wrap a towel around your calf and grasp both ends if you can't reach your leg with your hands). Pull your leg gently towards you, keeping it straight, to feel a stretch down the back of your leg. Flex your foot to increase intensity. Hold each leg for 10 seconds.

 2 ### GLUTE STRETCH
Lie on your back with your knees bent and feet flat on the floor. Raise both feet off the floor as you bend your left leg and place your left ankle just above your right knee. Grasp your right leg on either side with both hands (or use a towel to help), and gently pull it towards you. You should feel a stretch in your left glute. Hold for 10 seconds, then lower and repeat on the other side.

 3 ### QUADRICEPS STRETCH
Lie on your stomach, flex your right leg and take hold of your ankle with your right hand. If you can't reach, use a towel to help you. Resting your head on your left hand, press your right hip into the floor to feel a stretch along the front of your thigh. Keep your thighs pressed together throughout the stretch. Hold for 10 seconds, then swap legs.

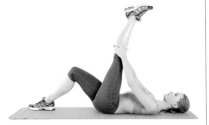

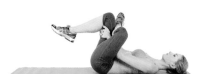

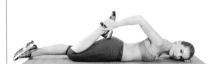

 4 ### CALF STRETCH
Step your right leg back, bending at your left knee, with both feet pointing forwards. Place your hands on your left thigh. Straighten your right leg, pressing your heel into the floor. Hold for 10 seconds, then swap sides.

 5 ### TRICEPS STRETCH
Standing with knees slightly bent and tummy in, lift your right arm and bend it behind your head. Push your right elbow gently with your left hand and try to reach between your shoulder blades. Stretch each arm for 10 seconds.

 6 ### CHEST STRETCH
Stand with your feet hip-width apart and knees soft. With your arms straight, take them out to the sides, then behind you, keeping your shoulders down. Feel a stretch across your chest. Hold for 10 seconds.

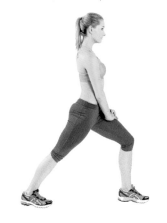

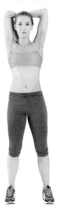

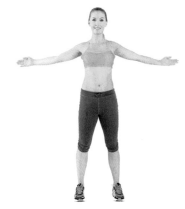

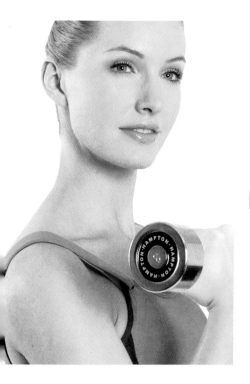

YOUR SIX-WEEK PLAN

This programme will help you ensure you get the results you want in time for the big day

The six-week plan opposite is perfect if you're a beginner or intermediate exerciser, as it steers you progressively from doing three workouts in the first week to five workouts in the sixth.

If you're a more advanced exerciser who trains regularly, skip to week four, then maintain the maximum five-workouts-a-week rhythm. You could also increase the weight of your dumbbells, working up to doing the progressions offered for each exercise, or upping the length of your cardio sessions.

THE PLAN EXPLAINED

Follow the training plan as closely as possible for optimum results.

MAIN WORKOUT DAYS
On the days marked 'Main workout', warm up, perform the eight exercises

from the main workout in order, then do the cool-down.

TARGET WORKOUT DAYS
On designated 'Target workout' days, warm up, then perform up to a maximum of three different Target workout circuits, followed by a cool-down. If you only have one problem area that you're concerned about, only do the relevant Target workout. These days are flexible, and the length of the overall workout can be as short or as long as you need it to be.

LONG CARDIO DAYS
Your 'Long cardio' days take the form of a 'steady state' cardio session (see the Cardio section on page 44 if you need a reminder about different types of cardio). Depending on your fitness levels, choose an activity such as walking, jogging, cycling or swimming and do it for the prescribed amount of time. You must also perform a warm-up and cool-down

either side of the prescribed length of your cardio session.

SHORT CARDIO SESSIONS
'Short cardio' sessions – added onto your Target workout days later on in the programme – are all about interval training. They are shorter, but feature quick bursts of intense activity at levels you wouldn't be able to sustain over a longer cardio session. You won't need to warm up if you do the Short cardio session immediately after your Target workout, but you will need to cool down afterwards, in addition to the prescribed length of the cardio session.

REST DAYS
On your rest days, don't do any intense exercise, but still try to do as much moderate activity as possible to maximise calorie burning. Take the stairs instead of the escalator or lift, walk or cycle to work and go for walks in your lunch break or at the end of the day.

WEEK	MON	TUES	WED	THURS	FRI	SAT	SUN
ONE	Main workout	REST	Target workout	REST	Long cardio (25 mins)	REST	REST
WRITE IN WHAT YOU DO HERE							
TWO	Main workout	Target workout	REST	Long cardio (30 mins)	Main workout	REST	REST
WRITE IN WHAT YOU DO HERE							
THREE	Main workout	Target workout	REST	Long cardio (35 mins)	Main workout	REST	REST
WRITE IN WHAT YOU DO HERE							
FOUR	Main workout	Target workout, plus 10 mins short cardio	Long cardio (40 mins)	REST	Main workout	Target workout, plus 12 mins short cardio	REST
WRITE IN WHAT YOU DO HERE							
FIVE	Long cardio (45 mins)	Main workout	Target workout, plus 15 mins short cardio	REST	Main workout	Target workout, plus 17 mins short cardio	REST
WRITE IN WHAT YOU DO HERE							
SIX	Long cardio (50 mins)	Main workout	Target workout, plus 20 mins short cardio	REST	Main workout	Target workout, plus 22 mins short cardio	REST
WRITE IN WHAT YOU DO HERE							

DON'T TRAIN ON REST DAYS – OVERTRAINING CAN LEAD TO INJURY AND ILLNESS

{ *Congratulations on completing your six-week plan! Keep progressing your workouts by increasing the weight of your dumbbells, working up to the progressive exercises or lengthening your cardio sessions.* }

Chart your
PROGRESS

Stay on target to be your beautiful best by tracking your weekly progress

There's nothing more motivating than being able to see the changes in your body shape and fitness as you begin to lose weight and get fitter. So before you start your six-week shape up, weigh or measure yourself and log your vital statistics in the chart below. Then weigh in and re-measure your stats every week on Mondays – first thing in the morning is best. Stick to this plan and you should start to notice a big difference in your measurements by week three, if not a little bit sooner – so there's no excuse to give up!

MEASURE YOUR WEIGHT LOSS
It's not just the scales that tell you how you're shaping up –in fact, they can be deceptive. Muscle weighs more than fat, so to get an idea of how slim and toned you're getting, it's best to measure your vital stats as well as weighing yourself. Here's what you need to measure and how to do it:
BUST Measure around the widest part of your bust, across your nipples.

WAIST Relax your tummy and take your measurement around your belly button.
HIPS Take your measurement around the widest part of your hips.
THIGH Measure your right thigh a quarter of the way down from your hip.

MEASURE YOUR FITNESS
As the weight comes off, you'll also be getting fitter. You can measure this by taking your resting heart rate, which should fall as you get fitter. It's a good idea to measure your resting heart rate once a week. To do this, simply take your

WEIGHT-LOSS CHART

Add your vital statistics each week and celebrate the results!

	WEEK 1	WEEK 2	WEEK 3	WEEK 4	WEEK 5	WEEK 6
WEIGHT						
BUST						
WAIST						
HIPS						
THIGHS						

RESTING HEART RATE

WEEK 1	
WEEK 2	
WEEK 3	
WEEK 4	
WEEK 5	
WEEK 6	

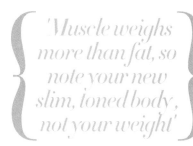

pulse, either on your wrist or your neck. Count how many beats there are in 15 seconds then multiply the result by four to find out your resting heart rate. Make a note of the number and, as you become fitter, you should see this number reduce. That's because your heart becomes more powerful and reduces the amount of beats it produces per minute.

Make sure you also log the results of your fitness tests on page 38 and 39 of this book, to measure your cardio fitness, flexibility and core strength.

FITNESS TESTS

Add your results each week and rejoice at your improvements!

	WEEK 1	WEEK 2	WEEK 3	WEEK 4	WEEK 5	WEEK 6
RUN TEST						
SIT-AND-REACH TEST						
SIT-UP TEST						

KEEP AT IT!
Don't panic if your fitness tests results are lower than you'd like at first. It doesn't matter if you record zero in the sit-up test or your cardio fitness is below average. Very soon you'll be making huge fitness gains and your motivation will get a massive boost when you see how far you've come.

Directory

FITNESS CLOTHING

ADIDAS
adidas.com
00800 378 74737

ASICS
asics.co.uk
01925 241041

CASALL
casall.co.uk
01458 274557

DOUNLIMITED
dounlimited.com

FREDDY
freddy.com
020 7836 5291

FROM CLOTHING
fromclothing.com
01404 510518

LESSBOUNCE
lessbounce.com
01985 851880

LET YOUR BODY BREATHE
letyourbodybreathe.com
020 7193 6342

LULULEMON
lululemon.co.uk
0800 783 9249

MANUKA
manukalife.com
020 7371 7878

MOVING COMFORT
movingcomfort.co.uk

NEW BALANCE
newbalance.co.uk
0808 101 2828

NIKE
store.nike.com

NO BALLS
noballs.co.uk
01638 570387

ON RUNNING
on-running.com

PANACHE
panache-lingerie.com
0845 270 6222

PINEAPPLE
pineapple.uk.com

REEBOK
reebok.com
0800 305 050

ROHAN
rohan.co.uk
0800 840 1412

RONHILL
ronhill.com
0161 366 5020

SHEACTIVE
sheactive.co.uk
0845 094 9434

SHOCK ABSORBER
shockabsorber.co.uk
0500 362 430

SKECHERS
skechers.co.uk
01707 624 772

STRIDERS EDGE
stridersedge.co.uk

STUDIO2
dwsports.com

SWEATY BETTY
sweatybetty.com
0800 169 3889

USA PRO
sportsdirect.com

VAUDE
vaude.co.uk
01665 510660

WELLICIOUS
wellicious.com
020 7221 3300

ZAGGORA
zaggora.com
07537 404575

ZOCA
sheactive.co.uk/zoca

FITNESS KIT

GARMIN.COM/UK
garmin.com/uk

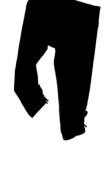

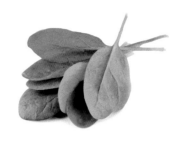

HAB DIRECT
habdirect.co.uk
01926 816100

OMRON
omronhealthcare.co.uk
0870 750 2771

PHYSICAL COMPANY
physicalcompany.co.uk
01494 769222

PHYSIO ROOM
physioroom.com

SUUNTO
suunto.co.uk
020 3608 0534

YOGA-MAD
yogamad.com
01386 859555

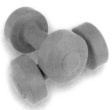

FOOD AND SUPPLEMENTS

AGAVE SYRUP
goodnessdirect.co.uk
0871 871 6611

BEAR
bearnibbles.co.uk
020 7183 0621

BEOND
pulsing.co.uk/beond-bars
01452 728900

BLISS
pulsin.co.uk/bliss-bar

BOUNCE
bouncefoods.com
0845 838 2579

BRITISH DIETETIC ASSOCIATION
bda.uk.com
0121 200 8080

CHERRYGOOD
cherrygood.com
020 7251 9924

CLIF
clifbar.co.uk

EAT NATURAL
eatnatural.co.uk
01787 479123

G.H.CRETORS
ghcretors.com

GOOD HEMP
goodwebsite.co.uk

HALE AND HEARTY
halenhearty.co.uk
020 7616 8427

HIGH 5
highfive.co.uk
01530 835873

INFINITY
infinityfoodsretail.co.uk
01273 603563

MAXITONE
maxitone.com
01442 244330

NAIRNS
nairns-oatcakes.com
0131 620 7000

NAKD
naturalbalancefoods.co.uk
0845 862 5340

9 BAR
9-bar.co.uk
01490 412297

NOSH DETOX
Noshdetoxdelivery.com
0845 257 6674

PURE PACKAGE
purepackage.com
020 7720 3250s

RAW HEALTH
rawhealth.uk.com
020 8547 2775

REFLEX
reflex-nutrition.com
01273 303817

RUDE HEALTH
rudehealth.com
0845 465 7833

SOLGAR
solgar.co.uk
01442 890355

THE FOOD DOCTOR
thefooddoctor.com
020 7792 6720

THE VILLAGE BAKERY
village-bakery.com
01768 898437

TREK
naturalbalancefoods.co.uk
0845 862 5340

VITABIOTICS
vitabiotics.com
020 8955 2662

XYLITOL
goodnessdirect.co.uk

BEAUTY

AVEDA
aveda.co.uk
0800 054 2979

BEAUBRONZ
beaubronz.co.uk
020 8788 7770

BLISS
blissworld.co.uk
0808 100 4151

CLINIQUE
clinique.co.uk
0800 054 2666

DECLÉOR
decleor.co.uk

DR HAUSCHKA
drhauschka.co.uk
01386 791 022

ELEMIS
elemis.com
0117 316 1888

FAKEBAKE
fakebake.co.uk
0844 856 5758

FAMOUS DAVE
famousdave.co.uk
01256 698 100

FANTASY TAN
0845 129 8431
fantasytan.co.uk

GREEN PEOPLE
greenpeople.co.uk
01403 740350

KÉRASTASE
kerastase.co.uk

LIZ EARLE
uk.lizearle.com
01983 813913

NEAL'S YARD REMEDIES
nealsyardremedies.com
0845 262 3145

ORGANIC PHARMACY
theorganicpharmacy.com
0844 800 8399

ORGANIC SURGE
organicsurge.com
01955 606061

ORIGINS
origins.co.uk
0800 054 2888

PHILIP KINGSLEY
philipkingsley.co.uk
020 7237 7100

SCHWARZKOPF
schwarzkopf.co.uk

SPATOPIA
sainsburys.co.uk

ST.TROPEZ
st-tropez.com
020 7845 6330

FITNESS

BIKRAM YOGA
bikramyoga.co.uk

BODY CONTROL PILATES
bodycontrolpilates.com
020 7636 8900

BRITISH WHEEL OF YOGA
bwy.org.uk
01529 306851

PILATES FOUNDATION
pilatesfoundation.com
020 7033 0078

PT FOLDER
ptfolder.com

RUN BRITAIN
runbritain.com

THE REGISTER OF EXERCISE PROFESSIONALS
exerciseregister.org

WOMEN'S SPORT AND FITNESS FOUNDATION
wsff.org.uk
02072731740

YOGA ALLIANCE
yogaalliance.co.uk

ZUMBA FITNESS
zumba.com

BRIDAL

COAST
coast-stores.com

BRILLIANT INC.
brilliantinc.co.uk

FIGLEAVES
figleaves.com
08444 932 932

IRRESISTIBLE HEADDRESSES
irresistibleheaddresses.com

LOVE ME DO BRIDES
lovemedobrides.com
01932 221 325

RAINBOW CLUB
rainbowclub.co.uk
01392 207 030

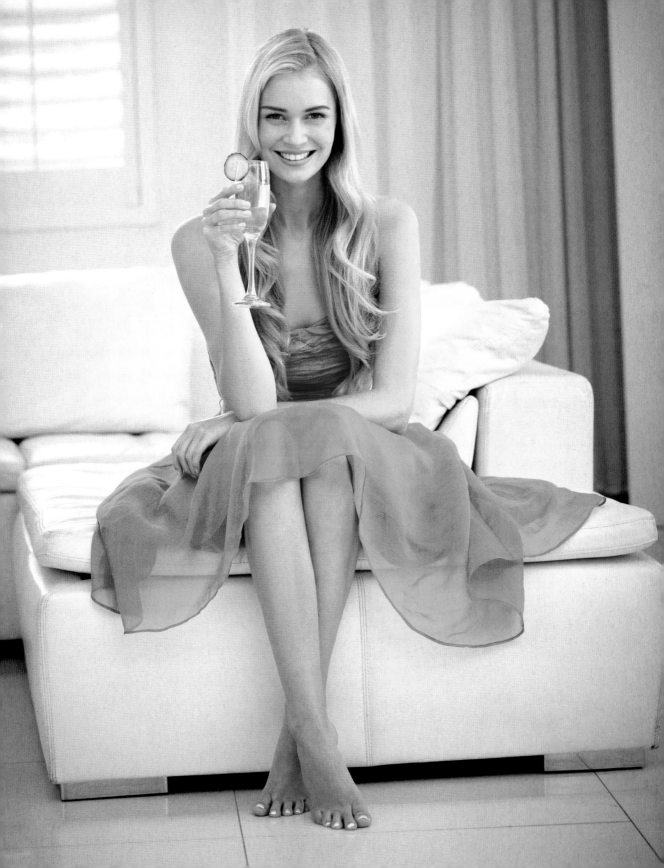

Happy WEDDING DAY!

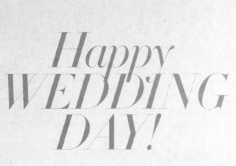

By the time you read this, you're hopefully well on your way to becoming the beautiful bride you've always wanted to be. If you've followed the exercise and healthy eating plans, plus our advice for getting gorgeous and staying relaxed, you should already be feeling fitter, healthier, happier, more self-assured, and ready to dazzle your guests on your special day.

Now it's time to enjoy the results of your hard work. Congratulations!

GET IN TOUCH

We'd love to hear how you get on and see the reults of your bridal shape-up makeover! Talk to us, and others doing the bridal shape-up plan, at facebook.com/HandFmagazine to share your achievements, ask for advice or swap inspiration with other readers.

CLOTHING: Coast dress, £250 (coast-stores.com). The Way You Look Tonight tiara, price on request.